VITALIZING
LONG-TERM CARE

Stuart F. Spicker, Ph.D., is Professor of Community Medicine and Health Care at the University of Connecticut School of Medicine in Farmington. He received his doctoral degree in philosophy from the University of Colorado. He is coeditor of the book series, *Philosophy and Medicine,* and coeditor of *Aging and the Elderly: Humanistic Perspectives in Gerontology.* He has been visiting professor of medical ethics at the Medizinische Hochschule Hannover in the Federal Republic of Germany, and served as Program Associate with the Technology Assessment and Risk Analysis Group at the National Science Foundation (1982–83).

Stanley R. Ingman, Ph.D., is Associate Professor of Family and Community Medicine at the University of Missouri School of Medicine, Columbia. He received his doctoral degree in sociology from the University of Pittsburgh. He was formerly Assistant Professor of Community Medicine and Health Care at the University of Connecticut School of Medicine, Farmington. He is coeditor with A. Thomas of *Topias and Utopias in Health.* He is also the author of numerous articles concerning the provision of geriatric care. In 1983, he was visiting professor at the Institut de Médecine Sociale et Préventive of the Université de Genève studying geriatric care systems in Switzerland.

VITALIZING LONG-TERM CARE

THE TEACHING NURSING HOME AND OTHER PERSPECTIVES

Stuart F. Spicker, Ph.D.
Stanley R. Ingman, Ph.D.
Editors

Foreword by Robert N. Butler, M.D.

SPRINGER PUBLISHING COMPANY
New York

To my wonderful Aunt Etta who is living alone in Los Angeles; she is not in a nursing home. Quite recently she began to draw and paint. Her brother, Phil Goldfaden, also lives alone in New Jersey; he too is still on his own and able to care for himself, though both worry a bit about the future and their health—but who doesn't?

S.F.S.

Springer Publishing Company, Inc.
200 Park Avenue South
New York, New York 10003

84 85 86 87 88 / 10 9 8 7 6 5 4 3 2 1

Library of Congress Cataloging in Publication Data

Main entry under title:
Vitalizing long-term care.

Bibliography: p. Includes index.
1. Aged—Care and hygiene. 2. Nursing home care. I. Spicker, Stuart F.
II. Ingman, Stanley R. [DNLM: 1. Long term care. 2. Geriatrics—
Education. 3. Nursing homes. WT 30 V837]
RA564.8.V58 1984 362.1'6'0973 84-1220
ISBN 0-8261-4570-1

Printed in the United States of America

Contents

Contributors

RUTH STUMPE BRENT, Ph.D., is Assistant Professor of Housing and Interior Design, College of Home Economics, University of Missouri at Columbia, Missouri.

RUTH CAMPBELL, M.S.W., is Senior Social Worker, Turner Geriatric Clinic, University of Michigan Hospital, Ann Arbor, Michigan.

ARTHUR L. CAPLAN, Ph.D., is Associate for the Humanities, The Hastings Center, Hastings-on-Hudson, New York.

DONALD O. COWGILL, Ph.D., is Professor Emeritus of Sociology, University of Missouri at Columbia, Missouri.

SALLY A. GADOW, Ph.D., R.N., is Associate Professor of Medical Humanities, Institute for the Medical Humanities, University of Texas Medical Branch, Galveston, Texas.

BERNICE HALBUR, Ph.D., is Assistant Professor of Sociology, School of Social and Behavioral Sciences, University of Alabama at Birmingham, Alabama.

THOMAS HALPER, Ph.D., is Professor of Political Science, Baruch College of the City University of New York, New York City.

STANLEY R. INGMAN, Ph.D., is Associate Professor of Social and Behavioral Science, School of Medicine, University of Missouri at Columbia, Missouri.

JEANIE S. KAYSER-JONES, Ph.D., is Associate Professor, Department of Family Health Care, School of Nursing, and Department of Epidemiology and International Health, School of Medicine, University of California at San Francisco, California.

PHYLLIS KULTGEN, Ph.D., is Assistant Research Professor, Center on Aging Studies, University of Missouri at Kansas City, Missouri.

IAN R. LAWSON, M.D., F.R.C.P., (Edinburgh) and F.A.C.P. is Professor of Community Medicine and Health Care (Geriatrics), School of Medicine, University of Connecticut Health Center, Farmington, Connecticut.

RICHARD A. LUSKY, Ph.D., is Assistant Professor of Community Medicine and Health Care (Sociology), School of Medicine, University of Connecticut, Health Center, Farmington, Connecticut.

CAROL L. PANICUCCI, Ph.D., R.N., is Assistant Professor of Nursing, School of Nursing, University of Wisconsin at Madison, Wisconsin.

FREDRICK T. SHERMAN, M.D., M.Sc., is Associate Professor of Clinical Geriatrics and Adult Development and of Clinical Medicine, Mount Sinai School of Medicine, Mount Sinai Medical Center, New York City.

STUART F. SPICKER, Ph.D., is Professor of Community Medicine and Health Care (Philosophy), School of Medicine, University of Connecticut Health Center, Farmington, Connecticut.

MICHAEL J. STOTTS, M.Ed., C.A.S., is Assistant Professor, Department of Internal Medicine, University of Nebraska Medical Center, Omaha, Nebraska.

KATHLEEN M. WOODWARD, Ph.D., is Associate Professor of English, University of Wisconsin at Milwaukee, Wisconsin.

MILDRED ZIMMERMAN, Ph.D., is a social worker in the Aging Department, Prairie View, Inc., a psychiatric hospital and mental health center, Wichita, Kansas.

Foreword

If over one million Americans were made homeless by a major disaster such as a flood, the immediate generosity of the public would be obvious. Unfortunately, over one million individuals living in American nursing homes have not enjoyed the degree of public and professional concern that is warranted.

It is time for a major move in long-term care. There must be a vitalization of the nursing home as an academic center. It is essential that medical, nursing, and allied health students have effective teaching experience in a quality nursing home environment. It is imperative that scientific inquiry center upon the many profound debilities to be observed among the residents of nursing homes. It is necessary that services in nursing homes be enhanced in quality and expanded in type to go far beyond the walls of the nursing home itself.

One way to mobilize our nation's resources to meet the needs for innovation and reform in nursing home care is the creation of a national commission on long-term care insurance composed of an independent body of outstanding persons from all walks of life devoted to a consolidation and review of contemporary knowledge, followed by the development of recommendations and an active plan to implement them. Such an effort will necessarily involve a call for reforms in reimbursement payments under Medicare, Medicaid and private insurance to practitioners, hospitals, and nursing homes.

For such a commission to accomplish its mission, it would have to turn to books such as this, which provide both the concepts and the knowledge base essential to the task. The topics covered are appropriately wide-ranging, from policy issues to the humanities, and from the creative arts to philosophy and clinical geriatric education.

Robert N. Butler, M.D.
The Mount Sinai Medical Center
New York City

Introduction

Unreflectively, the editors of *Vitalizing Long-term Care* originally chose the word "*re*vitalizing" to signal the title of this anthology; they themselves failed to observe that the typical American nursing home was, in fact, never "vitalized" in the first place. The editors' oversight perhaps makes it all the more important that the reader appreciate the need to vitalize these long-term care institutions. For it is one of the main theses of this collection that this is a propitious time to introduce the model of the teaching nursing home in long-term care settings which, at present, accommodate 1.3 million elderly residents in the United States.

Indeed, since this was written, the Mount Sinai Medical Center of the City University of New York has established the first Department of Geriatrics and Adult Development in the United States, which will function *within* the School of Medicine alongside other departments, like internal medicine, family medicine, and pediatrics. This event in itself constitutes a radical innovation in geriatric and gerontological education for students of medicine. Numerous, if not all, long-term care facilities which presently serve as the home of these elderly citizens are sitting dormant, awaiting the influx of students who one day will be socialized into the various health professions—not just medicine, but nursing, social work, the numerous allied health professions, such as rehabilitation and nutrition science, dentistry, pharmacy, and social services. This volume, then, is designed for the many students and faculty who, in time, will spend a good deal of their professional lives learning about aging *within* the long-term care institution in the context of the teaching nursing home. To be sure, not all of these institutions will be the recipients of these students, apprentices, and faculty from the health professions, but the hope is that—of the 126 schools of medicine in the United States—many will establish formal educational and teaching programs within these institutions and if not *re*vitalize them, then at least add an innovative vitality to the institutions.

While aging policy has not been directly informed by our most sophisticated vision or understanding of older adults' desires or needs, there is a growing consensus that as a society we ought to work toward that end. In Part I, Thomas Halper, Arthur Caplan, Stuart Spicker, Michael Stotts, and Jeanie Kayser-Jones raise important theoretical and political issues which require our attention if the nursing home is to become part of the mainstream of the social and clinical service delivery arena—one in which medical students, for example, may learn the clinical skills of their profession.

Halper, Stotts, and Kayser-Jones raise three issues which are important for geriatric and gerontological health professionals and activists, and they demand a creative response: (1) the proper role of medicine in response to an aging population; (2) the level of organizational sophistication required to properly administer long-term care institutions; and (3) the nature of the financial incentives germane to the latter two. In addition, an *active* response is required, otherwise nursing home and geriatric care will remain nothing more than a seasonal crisis—oscillating between avoidance and neglect of the aged. Physicians will continue to be uncommitted, and financial doom and gloom for Medicare and Medicaid will be more than a theoretical possibility.

For Halper (Chapter 1), one issue is whether age-based services, transfer payments, and tax expenditures for the aged account for the declining status and decreasing autonomy of the aged. A realistic understanding and appreciation of dependency among the aged in our society is an appropriate place to begin a critical analysis of the nursing home as a social and health-care institution. For too long, appeals to improve the nursing home have had to confront the claim that we cannot afford any reform because the burden of current nursing home costs is already overwhelming.

The reader is asked to question his or her conception of medicine, the relationship between aging and disease, and the "biology of aging." Much of the gerontological and activist community has sought to disentangle the phenomenon of aging from the notion of disease. Arthur L. Caplan (Chapter 2) asks the crucial question: Is aging a disease? Caplan realizes that most persons in our society would be loathe to learn that aging is properly classified as a disease. Yet, he answers that the characterization of aging as a "natural" or "normal" process rests on faulty biological analysis. He admits that good arguments might be made against excluding aging from the purview of medicine, but they cannot be made on the grounds that aging is natural. As Caplan observes, the medical professions and thus medical students have difficulty becoming interested in the various conditions mentioned above, because of their less-than-straightforward relationship to the phenomenon of disease.

Stuart Spicker (Chapter 3) argues that our concept of human aging is confused. Spicker questions the biogerontologists, who focus their attention on deteriorative processes, decreased viability, and increased vulnerability. Persons are not a collection of cells or organelles, nor is human aging and growing old simply the inability to reproduce. He challenges the biologists' claim that they study the biology of aging. Instead, he shows that they focus on the human life span, the prevention of disease, and cellular processes which function as 'markers' of aging at the micro level. For Spicker, human aging is a personal process which cannot be captured by our typical chronometric notion of time. He therefore appears to disagree with Caplan's thesis that aging is a disease.

Focusing on the broader policy issues, Stotts (Chapter 4) calls for reform of the long-term care "system" if we are to be successful at the micro level, that is, the individual nursing home. Isolating nursing homes from the universities, their health professional schools of medicine, nursing, social work, and local hospitals, as well as community mental health centers, must eventually cease. Nursing homes must soon begin to establish alternative care programs as additional means of providing opportunities for offering good services to their "clients," that is, *residents* in their community. Stotts employs the term "client-centered policy" to describe a long-term care system which points to a shift in orientation. He raises key questions: How do we begin to reorganize our local care system? Can care-system building go on within a context of competition between proprietary interests? Can we temper the "take charge" tendency of full-time care systems (like nursing homes) by allowing *non-professional* friends and relatives to take on a caring role? Can hospitals, nursing homes, and especially home-care institutions learn to deal with independent clients and their supporters who wish to define needs in their own terms? Are we ever going to analyze and compare *total* system expenditures instead of focusing on misleading comparisons of nursing and home-care costs?

The concept of a total-care system almost defies definition and makes cross-national comparisons a rocky road at least. Nevertheless, Jeanie Kayser-Jones's (Chapter 5) comparative work on Scotland and the United States serves to dramatically challenge U.S. nursing home research, such as Bruce Vladeck's *Unloving Care: The Nursing Home Tragedy* (1980). She confronts those who try to sell the "sameness" among U.S. nursing homes as "normal," unchangeable, or the best that may be possible. Reform in either the United States or Scotland will not and has not come through quick fixes. Rather, structural reforms which reward nurse and physician involvement is a more viable starting point. In the U.S. context it may mean rearranging incentives, for example, decreasing incentives for involvement in other traditional medical specialties, such as radiology, surgery, or other more lucrative subspecialties.

What strikes numerous visitors to Scotland is how unaware geriatricians there are of the structural elements of their own social and medical care system. They typically point to the process of quality recruitment and selection of professionals as the major precondition for excellence.

The notion of introducing a geriatrician as a care provider, working alongside other health providers with gerontological training, is hotly debated in the United States today. Stresses and strains with respect to the role of the geriatrician exist in Europe, and even in Britain. Nevertheless, the demographic "geriatric momentum" continues to exert steady pressure on the delivery system and calls for an improved professional response.

Introducing Part II, Ian Lawson (Chapter 6) is clearly not sanguine when he considers the introduction of geriatric education into the long-term care arena—given that there are so many conflicts and antitheses underlying quality geriatric practice, and the current norms and rules that govern how professionals are expected to practice clinical medicine. He argues that the mere addition of courses or clerkships in geriatrics in various schools of medicine may not have a truly significant impact on practice and performance. He addresses four major contextual or structural weaknesses: (1) professionals tend to focus on acute or curative medical care; (2) the present financial incentive system favors provider priorities at the expense of meeting patient care needs; (3) there exists an administratively nonintegrated system, where each institution relentlessly seeks to fill its beds, capture third-party eligibility, or add one more item of service to enlarge its domain. This is clearly not a social world where team or institutional coordination comes easily; and finally, (4) medical faculties, with their increasingly narrow clinical and biological focus, feel extremely uneasy in discussions of multiproblem-oriented "holism" germane to the clinical care of older patients.

Aware of a geriatric context of structural and attitudinal antitheses, as Dr. Lawson describes them, Dr. Fredrick T. Sherman (Chapter 7) critically and carefully outlines the process of designing a teaching nursing home or a long-term care system in which to train medical students. A review of the literature reveals that attitudes among medical students become somewhat more positive with respect to geriatric practice once they are exposed to nursing home care. However, students seem to profit more from exposure to the entire range of clinical services which support the aged. Sherman reviews many topics and content areas which can be taught within the nursing home itself. Examples of this include differentiation between normal aging and disease; rehabilitation of patients who suffered stroke, arthritis, or who require hip and amputation care; diagnostic and therapeutic approaches to a variety of communication disorders; complex multisystem clinical decision making; appropriate placement of patients; team care and pharmacokinetics and pharmacodynamics. But in which years and under which formats should the nursing home experience be introduced into the curriculum? Answer: throughout the four-year program! With some creativity and care, the Introduction to Medicine, and the History and Physical Examination programs can, for example, help to create and foster an initial and positive geriatric attitude and skill-formation experience. A geriatric clerkship introduced in the third or fourth year is still another relatively unexplored opportunity. This author warns, however, that present financial incentive structures, which encourage short and infrequent visits to the local nursing home, may have to be reformed at the academic level as well as at the community level before the truly functional academic teaching nursing home can become a reality.

According to Sherman, a good deal of general geriatric medicine and care can be taught well in the single-level nursing home. This is possible because nursing home residents tend to exhibit multiple pathology, and this serves as a basis for teaching medical students. Secondly, knowledge gained within nursing homes is widely applicable to other independent elderly.

To be effective, Sherman maintains that three issues must be directly addressed: (1) Who will teach? (2) What will be taught? (3) Is the nursing home a credible education site? Monitoring systems, staff conferences, and continuing education are activities which need to be improved in order to augment services as well as teaching capacities in the nursing home. Caring physician teachers—even if not the academic élite—are preferred to typically disinterested academics. Sherman argues that direct student precepting by faculty at the bedside will unquestionably attract students. Preparing students and staff to appreciate various expectations and roles will also play an important educational function.

Dr. Sherman also notes that geriatric medicine must soon focus attention on functional assessment and not just diagnosis. Carol

Panicucci (Chapter 8) examines the question more directly: What is the conceptual base for the use of functional assessment in clinical geriatric practice? As she observes, terms like *functional abilities* and *functional assessment* are subject to different interpretations. The power of this approach is located in four factors: (1) functional independence is a relevant concern for all clients; (2) many elderly think in terms of health or functional status, as opposed to the language of disease labels; (3) functional assessment is easily understood by both professionals and clients and increases communication; and (4) functional assessment is more likely to secure the participation of the client into his or her own therapeutic plan. Panicucci argues that a functional approach which focuses on the patient's coping abilities is more appropriate than the typical problem-oriented assessment with its focus on morbidity.

To clarify the concept *long-term care system,* Stanley Ingman and Bernice Halbur (Chapter 9) encourage us to take a closer look at the typical community hospital in terms of its service goals, as well as its educational role within geriatric practice. A combination of negative attitudes and poor care seem to demand some sort of compelling response. Moreover, each phase of care requires reform: (1) the preadmission phase; (2) in-patient care; and (3) the discharge process. A review of these phases can redefine the meaning of so-called "standard clinical practice for the frail aged."

Opening Part III, Sally Gadow (Chapter 10) gently leads us into the topic by examining our historically changing vision of age and aging, as well as our militancy as it emerges in our will to reform geriatric medical education. Starting with the negative end of the spectrum—the view of aging as only a stage of dying—we move to a slightly more charitable view which elevates the elderly to underprivileged citizens so they may be the recipients of our beneficence. With the drive for geriatric medicine arises the view that aging is a unique human phenomenon. Finally, we are led to a view of the elderly as a cultural treasure, a repository of wisdom and an embodiment of history. Gadow also notes the negative value as well as the progressive impact of each new vision as it emerges. As she indicates, there is *no* one correct way to regard aging when we attend to the so-called "facts." Most sharply, she formulates the important question: How can the humanities (e.g., literature, philosophy, history, the fine and creative arts) contribute to a geriatric curriculum? At the personal level, Gadow discusses how the humanities can help develop an openness to and an appreciation of the many ways in which it is possible to experience aging. Policy issues with their intrinsic ethical components are yet another important set of concerns. Kathleen Woodward (Chapter 11) explores the role of literature in the geriatric context, and in our search for a more appropriate vision of aging. She describes Simone de Beauvoir's changing vision of aging and frailty from the writings *Coming of Age* and *A Very Easy Death*. Essentially, Beauvoir's was a transition from a vision of old age as "a dreaded decline" to a positive vision of the final days of frailty before death. She reinforces Gadow's point that philosophy and literature do not primarily function to show us our errors or to move us in the "right" direction. Literature surely leads us to appreciate the ambiguous nature and character of our existence. Finally, Woodward reviews Bernard Berenson's diary, *Sunset and Twilight*. Beside his frustration with frailty, Berenson locates its redemption: (1) we see more clearly than ever before; (2) our contentment with merely "being" is made salient; (3) we are witness to the love of others in dependency. One is reminded of Beauvoir's belief that in old age we should continue to define ourselves by *our* action.

Ruth Campbell (Chapter 12) describes one process whereby aged, "nonprofessional" or lay writers, philosophers, and sociologists (unlike a Berenson or Beauvoir) reflect on the past, the present, and the nature of death. These lay women and men are members of a geriatric clinic. They come together to read their memoirs, their fictional works, their poetry, and their essays. She demonstrates that this process enables them to reveal more about their selves, their strengths, and their own identity. Campbell's discussion serves to extend Robert Butler's work on life review and the healing power of reminiscence. She also reviews the arguments of critics of gerontology's focus on reminiscence and life review. For example, is the world "over-medicalized" when Arthur Koestler suggests that "all creative activity is a kind of do-it-yourself therapy, an attempt to come to terms with traumatizing challenges"? As Campbell describes the people who attend these sessions, it is clear that there is a delightful mix of people and purposes, much as would be found in any social group or voluntary association. Personal problems, individual depression, value exploration, ethical questions, and current and historical themes, are all part of the social setting that allows these group sessions to flourish.

In Part IV, four institutional arenas are analyzed with respect to the ways they may be reformed: (1) nursing homes; (2) rehabilitation medicine; (3) mental health care; and (4) hospital care. Ruth Brent (Chapter 13), a designer and social scientist, asks us to be more creative about designing the various living spaces or dwellings we create, especially the nursing homes. She employs the Lawton and Nahemow "docility hypothesis" as the theoretical construct to initiate her argument: As health and competence decline, the elderly become more vulnerable to environmental influences. Elitist notions that designers, architects, and administrators should be the only persons involved in designing and building nursing homes is dispelled by Brent's analysis. Perhaps when future and present residents in various health care sectors become powerful and respected actors, then the entire range of fundamental concerns can be addressed, for example, privacy, personalization, temperature levels, lighting, and odors. It is not that other environments are devoid of these problems, but that the ability to change one's environment allows the human spirit to flourish, even when a particular home environment is extremely bleak. Brent offers a serious discussion to focus our attention on two central goals: (1) cultivation of public social space, and (2) cultivation of private spaces.

Richard Lusky (Chapter 14) also urges us to expand our vision on a more abstract plane. We are asked to try to comprehend the complex structural features in community care systems as they hinder or facilitate holistic health and social care delivery for the aged in our society. Lusky refers to the problems which are partially derived from a care system principally designed for the resolution of short-term acute health problems in otherwise healthy people. The struggle of the rehabilitation care movement in the United States provides many useful insights into the difficulties that the geriatric care movement of the 1970s has had to face and will continue to confront in the 1980s.

The central adjectival modifiers of the rehabilitation movement and the medical management of disability are important to recall: (1) comprehensive; (2) aggressive; (3) ongoing; (4) individualized; and (5) integrated. From Lusky's review of stroke and hip care patients, the existence of autonomous care institutions under a "free" market system is the most striking impediment to long-term stroke care. He views the recent expansion of federal programs in the field of aging with mixed feelings and asks: Will this expansion contribute to the kind of organizational environment which tends to increase or decrease fragmentation? His careful study of rehabilitation services suggests the conclusion that the availability and accessibility of the relevant health care services do not tend to guarantee their utilization.

Millie Zimmerman and Phyllis Kultgen (Chapter 15) shift our attention to the psychological environment which influences elderly experience in our society. In agreement with other contributors to the volume, these researchers conclude that our nosology and ways of talking about an elderly person's mental status need clarification *before* we begin to reorganize our care system; for example, there is confusion about terms like *mental health, mental illness,* and *mental disease*. Before discussing therapeutic interventions, the authors remind us that when a society is healthy its members have a greater opportunity to be healthy, that is, a positive social environment promotes healthy individuals. The underlying assumption is that an individual's identity and self-concept is shaped within group contexts. For example, social isolation for older women is a critical issue today, since nearly one-third of all women 65 years and older live alone.

Zimmerman and Kultgen offer a model for positive social support that fully comprehensive mental health programs might adopt. Components of this model include but are not limited to the following: (1) an elderly group; (2) the health professional as counselor; (3) the elderly's peers as counselors; (4) the family as counselors; (5) the clergy as counselors; and finally (6) personnel in the aging network as counselors. Some objections to the implementation of this model are also addressed. This essay seeks to make us aware that so often federal, state, or county planning bodies tend to slide almost unwittingly into narrow or unimaginative programs. These researchers boldly attempt to initiate a broader range of options.

In the closing memoir, Donald Cowgill (Chapter 16) writes as a gerontologist who approaches his own retirement. With a gentle balance between the past and present, he underscores a number of themes discussed by other contributors to this volume. First, Cowgill recalls his intellectual as well as his initial emotional reaction to the rhetorical question: Can we afford our aging population? His essay reveals how our affluent society has actually experienced a decline in the dependency ratio due to falling birth rates. Second, recalling that his mentor, Stuart Queen, treated aging as social pathology—much like unemployment or mental illness—Cowgill recounts with shock an earlier request that he speak to the topic, "Aging as a Social Disease." He then reviews the history of disengagement theory and reflects on the way the theory was co-opted to provide a convenient, naturalistic, scientific rationale for quiet retirement from the labor force. Custodial treatment and social isolation became quite easy to justify under this theory. Finally, Cowgill—along with his colleague Lowell Homes—raises the question: How has the status of the aged changed with the evolution to modern society? His response to this question provides a basis for designing service and educational programs which create fewer rather than more problems.

With various initiatives taken by federal agencies and private foundations, there is a good deal about which we may be somewhat optimistic. Recently, for example, impressive awards have been announced: The Geriatric Medicine Academic Award from both the National Institute on Aging (NIA) and the National Institute of Mental Health; support for Geriatric Research and Training Centers sponsored by the Veterans Administration; and most recently the Teaching/Nursing Home Grants sponsored by NIA as well as another set of Teaching/Nursing Home Grants to schools of nursing awarded by the Robert Wood Johnson Foundation. Those who would like to see improved geriatric care in the United States should be encouraged. However, a word of caution seems equally warranted.

Many geriatric clinicians and advocates of the aged have become disillusioned with the failure to properly implement the programs noted above. Put simply, they view the universities, researchers, and government officials as bastardizers of the original intent of these initiatives. "Bastardization" here means the manipulation of the programs and redirection of the funds to support more "traditional"— that is, biological—research under a new label which just happens to be "geriatric medicine." If the worry is a real one (and it is), we will come to discover that Teaching/Nursing Home proposals (TNH) are rejected when they emphasize the reorganization of care and stress gerontological research and clinical geriatric issues. Instead, we will find that TNH proposals are approved and funded when they stress "traditional" National Institutes of Health (NIH) research projects to be conducted by nongerontological researchers who earned credentials and reputations in other areas.

The Veterans Administration may by now have recognized the problem: Geriatric Research and Education Centers (GREC) which emphasize service, teaching, and research framed in a genuine geriatric orientation are now receiving stronger support, and GREC Centers which are more traditional in their orientation are responding to "gerontologize" their programs. Because the nursing schools are less likely to have an NIH organization, the Robert Wood Johnson Foundation Teaching/Nursing Home awards may have a better chance to vitalize the geriatric care sector. However, without a viable, clinically-oriented cadre of academic geriatric clinicians and researchers residing in our nation's schools of medicine, nursing home care will in all likelihood remain unaffected by these new federal programs.

If nursing-home care continues to remain a tertiary national concern, it is likely that nursing homes will remain underfunctional, nonprofessional custodial institutions. If nursing homes become defined as merely new places to locate indigent subjects for research carried out by university researchers, a grim assessment will remain for the year 2020 and beyond: Few nursing homes in the United States will be of high quality, will have clean and pleasant surroundings, well-prepared meals, a variety of activities, a staff to assist the residents in dressing and bathing, ample privacy for the residents, and first-rate medical and nursing services.

As today's young health professional students and faculty, and elderly residents with their midlife relatives in long-term care institutions, eventually find themselves interacting on a more continuous, daily, and intense level, one can only hope that by the end of this century and into the next, the words of Donald Cowgill will no longer serve as a description of the present state of affairs:

> The prestige and honor of the elderly compared with younger age groups has declined. Their disadvantage is psychological rather than life-threatening. It is nonetheless painful and humiliating.

It would be unfortunate if this anthology, in the end, is praised for being published some years ahead of its time.

Stuart F. Spicker
Stanley R. Ingman

Acknowledgments

As the complex projects which led to the completion and publication of this volume required the participation of a number of people in addition to the contributors, the editors would like to extend their personal gratitude to each of them.

In the initial phase of the project, we were assisted by the thoughtful and competent staff of the National Endowment for the Humanities. Richard Hedrich (now retired from the Endowment) and Carole Huxley assisted us in obtaining a Chairman's Grant under Special Programs (AP-20093-80-1491) to materially sustain the first conference entitled "Humanities in Gerontology and Geriatric Medicine: Toward a Further Integration." We are also grateful to Lorraine Schroeder, Susan Bernstein, Lynn Smith, and Joyce Wendell at the Endowment.

Mary O'Brien—at the time working at the Gerontological Institute of the University of Michigan—ably assisted in the work of the project, especially the "Humanities in Gerontology" section of the Annual Meeting of The Gerontological Society, which convened in San Diego, California, November 21–25, 1980.

Thanks are also extended to Professors Ronald Gottesman and Henry Clark III, respectively, of the Center for the Humanities, University of Southern California, who served as chairmen of the sessions, and enabled the initial conference to include very rewarding discussions following the formal presentations.

A second conference served to enable the editors to obtain additional contributions to the volume. During May 21–23, 1981, this joint conference was held at the University of Missouri at Columbia. With the support and assistance of Professor Patricia Morrow, Ph.D. (University of Missouri at Rolla), "Humanities, Social Science and Geriatric Education" convened cotemporaneously with her well-organized "The Meanings of Old Age."

This conference was materially supported by the Department of Family and Community Medicine (School of Medicine, University of Missouri at Columbia); The Research Council of the School of Medicine; The Graduate School; The Missouri Gerontological Institute and the Center for Aging Studies of the University of Missouri at Columbia.

Two additional federal awards provided material support: A Geriatric Curriculum Grant, awarded by the Bureau of Health Professions, Division of Medicine (HRA, DHHS), and an Aging Postdoctoral Program Award from the National Institute of Mental Health. We are especially grateful to Weldon Webb and the staff of the Office of Continuing Education and Extension for the Health Professions, School of Medicine at Columbia, who so ably resolved the logistical problems for the joint conference.

During the months this collection was in preparation, G. M. Fitzgerald and S. G. M. Engelhardt served the project as editorial assistants; without their dedication to the manuscript we would not have seen its publication. We also thank Ms. Carolyn A. Duca for her gracious typing assistance during the final stage of preparation of the manuscript.

The editors acknowledge with gratitude the many suggestions for improving the text which were offered by two conscientious readers: Richard Ratzan, M.D., and Kathleen Woodward, Ph.D.

Finally, we wish to extend our mutual appreciation to Robert N. Butler, M.D., Brookdale Professor of Geriatrics and Adult Development and Chairman of the Gerald and May Ellen Ritter Department of Geriatrics and Adult Development at Mount Sinai Medical Center, New York. Dr. Butler graciously contributed his Foreword despite his very demanding schedule. Some readers may recall that when Dr. Butler was Director of the National Institute on Aging, he initiated the concept of teaching nursing homes—institutions which would, in time, affiliate with universities and their schools—especially medicine, nursing, and social services. Dr. Butler is clearly the driving spirit behind this volume. We conclude by acknowledging his thoughts:

> As long as [geriatrics] lacks a solid research and training base, our programs will be chained to ineffective or partially effective methods of diagnosis, treatment, prevention, and rehabilitation, to procedures less efficient or more costly than need be, and to an arid intellectual and numbing emotional climate in long-term care. (*Aging Update*, NIA, n.d. Edited by M. A. Kurz and P. Jones. Information Office, U.S. DHHS (396), PHS, NIH.)

S.F.S.
S.R.I.

PART I
THEORETICAL AND POLITICAL IMPLICATIONS FOR AGING POLICY

1

Aging Policy in the Eighties: Second Thoughts on a Strategy that has Worked

THOMAS HALPER

"If it ain't broke," as Bert Lance used to say, "don't fix it." No one, I think, would suggest that the political strategy formulated and executed by the aged and their defenders over the past two decades is "broke." The current federal budget, like its recent predecessors, allocates nearly as much money to the elderly as to national defense.[1] Indeed, there are no fewer than 134 federal programs designed to assist the elderly. Disregarding inflation, public spending for retirement programs and tax benefits for the elderly doubled from 1969 to 1979 and will double again for 1979 to 1983. Even President Reagan's 1981 budget cuts project Social Security (old age and survivor pensions) and Medicare budgets at $275 billion per year in five years, a figure over fifty percent higher than current expenditures. This is hardly a record of failure.

Yet times change, and sometimes it is well to look a bit ahead to the future in the interest of not riding the same horse too long. It is in this spirit that I offer the following argument, not with certitude but rather in the hope that it may stir some profitable debate. The argument goes like this:

However understandable, the elderly's traditional demands for more age-based services, transfer payments, and tax expenditures raise three basic problems. They are founded upon an unrealistically gloomy reading of the aged's plight; they undermine the aged's demand for respect and autonomy; and they imperil the aged's credibility in an era of heightened economic insecurity and cutbacks in government social welfare programs. In the Reagan years, in short, a continuation of the strategy which has worked so brilliantly since the Johnson years may no longer be appropriate.

Let me try to expand on these points.

The demand by the aged for more services, transfer payments, and tax expenditures certainly *are* understandable, for the aged obviously constitute a most vulnerable stratum of the population. Even if an elder's health or financial circumstances seem perfectly adequate, there is always the possibility of sudden disastrous change from which recovery may prove only limited at best. Though such an eventuality may never occur or may be very late in coming, that it is perceived as an ever-present threat may itself be a source of anxiety.

Politically, also, demanding *more* is certainly understandable. Indeed, it is the staple technique of American interest groups from auto manufacturers to dairy farmers to labor unions to welfare rights organizations. For the elderly, so long neglected by government, loud complaints and demands were needed to get the official and public attention necessary to place their problems near the top of the political agenda. These complaints and demands continued in order to get key legislation passed and regulations adopted, and they continue today as a means of broadening and maintaining these benefits. And to the extent that the complaints and demands have succeeded in achieving these aims, they have reinforced the practice and encouraged other claimants with other constituencies to follow it. Thus, candidates, officeholders, journalists, talk show hosts, and vast numbers of ordinary citizens routinely declaim on the material and spiritual wretchedness of old age in America and on government's responsibility to alleviate the hardships. (Frequently, these remarks are prefaced by the assertion that "the problems of the American elderly have gone practically unnoticed,"[2] a statement so effectively refuted by its own repetition that one is reminded of Kerensky's sobriquet as "history's most famous forgotten man.")

While a significant proportion of the elderly do experience real economic problems, however, there can be no doubt that the rhetoric selling social programs and enhancing media drama has exaggerated the extent of the misery. A recent Harris poll, for instance, disclosed that while 68 percent of those under age 65 say that "not having enough money to live on" is "a very serious problem" for the elderly, only 17 percent of the elderly agree that this is true for themselves.[3] Government statistics themselves, in fact, have proven valuable allies in this exaggeration. According to government figures, for example, 15.1 percent of the elderly are poor.[4] These figures, however, are defined in terms of reported money income only. Consider what is left out: in-kind government programs (food stamps, Medicare, public housing, rent supplements, etc.); unreported income (gifts from family and friends, working "off the book" to avoid Social Security penalties, insurance settlements, lump sum inheritances); previously acquired assets (home, car, furnishings); and special tax benefits (double exemption on federal income tax, exemption of Social Security income and veterans and railroad retirement benefits from taxation, property tax relief granted in every state). Furthermore, government figures use the individual or family as the basic unit, not the household, although it is very common for elders to live together and remain unmarried in order to avoid losses in Social Security benefits and the marriage penalty in taxes. Finally, whereas the figures count as poor those who report little or no income (or even losses) because of farm or business losses or accelerated real estate depreciation, these persons are not in fact poor at all. One scholar found, when looking at the nation's total population, that the official method of calculation inflated the percentage of the poor in America by almost 400 percent.[5] There are good reasons for suspecting that poverty among the aged is also significantly overstated.

This is not to say, of course, that the aged are notable for their prosperity. In 1977, median family income for the elderly was only 57 percent of the national average and median income for elderly singles only 65 percent. There is less to these low percentages, however, than meets the eye. For the elderly are spared many of the expenses that the rest of society must pay: the elderly pay lower taxes, have fewer dependents to support, are less likely to have work-related expenses (like clothing and transportation) since most do not work, and are less likely to have mortgage expenses inasmuch as most own homes on which the mortgage has already been paid off.[6] And while the aged are more likely to be sick, the overwhelming majority are well. (Health expenses for persons over age 65 average 3.4 times greater than for those under age 65, but this is mostly offset by the government's paying nearly two-thirds of these costs.)

Selling always involves overselling, of course, but the exaggeration of the elderly's suffering has begun to exacerbate a pair of problems that may eventually render the strategy counterproductive. One problem is that the aged cannot be depicted as poor and suffering without also being consigned to a socially inferior status. The pity, compassion, and guilt that their complaints are designed to evoke identify them as helpless, and call upon society—through its coercive instrument, government,—to play the helper. But a class that assumes the role of the supplicant will always find it hard to be accepted by its suppliers as their equal.[7] In its opposition to long-standing protective legislation, the women's movement has evidenced some recognition that a choice must be made between demanding special benefits by dint of alleged frailties and demanding equal treatment by dint of alleged competence.[8] The day may not be far off when the elderly must make this choice too.

What is at stake here is not only society's perception of the aged, though it certainly makes an immense difference as to whether the aged are seen as "losers" and "has-beens" or as equals. For as one sociologist put it, "What man perceives as real is real in its consequences," and the consequences of widely held gerontophobic stereotypes are felt in innumerable personal interactions and decisions and in the public policy that to some extent mirrors public beliefs.

What is also at stake, however, is the elderly's perception of themselves. When an eminent gerontologist singled out self-esteem as the "linchpin of quality of life for the aged,"[9] he identified its importance as well. But if the aged acquiesce to the stigma of incompetence (or even inflict it upon themselves)—whatever the short-term political justification—they may be striking at their own sense of dignity and self-worth.

A second problem with exaggerating the troubles of the aged is that it weakens their credibility in an era of austerity. The Reagan administration has repeatedly declared that the only justification for receiving federal aid is demonstrable need. It is obvious that this policy is frequently honored mostly in the breach. But it is also obvious that programs—especially social programs—that do not meet this criterion will be vulnerable, and helping individuals because they are elderly rather than because they are needy may be increasingly difficult to defend. The Older American Act of 1965—"aging's Magna Carta"[10]—of course follows this principle precisely.

Already there are signs that programs that aid the elderly as a class, irrespective of need, are being questioned in ways that were unthinkable only a few years ago. There has been considerable talk, for example, of taxing Social Security benefits,[11] altering or abolishing their indexing arrangement,[12] lowering Social Security benefits for those with high lifetime earnings,[13] and abolishing the elderly's double income tax exemption.[14] Sharply reducing benefits for those retiring at age 62 has already been formally proposed and the House and Senate chairmen of the two chambers' respective Social Security subcommittees have advocated raising the age standard from 65 to 68.[15] Even before the 1980 election, President Carter's special adviser on aging chided the elderly for demanding a "selfish" share of special concessions and services, and suggested that this "could create resentment" on the part of younger taxpayers.[16]

These moves may be just the beginning. For as the elderly become steadily more numerous and their programs more expensive, the burden on the rest of society will become very heavy very quickly. In a confident time of economic expectations, this burden may be tolerated, but in a context of growing insecurity and anxiety, it is likely to seem unnecessary and unjust and "scrutiny will supplant sympathy."[17] With Social Security contributions often consuming a larger portion of an inflation-shrunken paycheck than federal or state income taxes, for example, an increasing number of workers will ask themselves why they should support a redistribution system that seems to be based more on age than on need. (Maximum annual payments zoomed from $20 in 1936 to $374.40 in 1970 to $1,587.67 in 1980 to a projected $3,410.55 in 1986.) Steadily lower worker-to-beneficiary ratios,[18] more aggressive demands for liberalized benefits, unemployment-induced shortfalls in payroll receipts, and the continuation of indexing can only add to the burden.

More broadly, consider the implications of President Reagan's budgetary strategy. About three-quarters of the budget is defined as "uncontrollable," meaning that it involves paying for prior fixed commitments (like the national debt) or entitlement programs that provide that, if individuals or state and local governments meet certain prescribed qualifying standards, they become entitled to federal aid. It is very difficult to control the "uncontrollables," and the Reagan administration has thus far approached them with great caution. But since much of the "controllable" portion of the budget goes for defense, an area which the administration is committed to enhance, there is not much in this portion that can be cut, either. Indeed, most of what can be cut probably has already been cut. This raises, therefore, the question of what will be cut in succeeding years. Clearly, social welfare entitlement programs, including those benefiting the elderly, will be obvious candidates for reductions.

What, then, should be done? It is always easier to identify problems than to propose solutions, but perhaps I can suggest two general approaches that seem to be on the ascendancy. One is increasingly to confine aid to the needy. The double tax exemption, for instance, benefits the elderly with adjusted gross incomes over $100,000 an

average of $553; the very poor—those with incomes under $3,000—
benefit to the tune of $4. It has been suggested, therefore, that the
exemption practice be dropped, in favor of progressively drawn or
equal tax credits, or simply discontinued altogether. Questions have
also been raised as to whether Medicare should continue to apply
without a means test. When, it is contended, over a billion dollars per
year is spent on health payments for elderly with annual incomes
exceeding $30,000, public funds are being senselessly substituted for
private funds.[19]

By diverting benefits from the non-needy to the needy—it is
argued—funds can be used with far more efficiency, the tax burden
can be kept within manageable proportions, and popular resentment
against the elderly can be curbed before a destructive backlash sets
in. In the long run, say advocates of this view—say, in 60 years when
nearly 20 percent of the nation will be over age 65—these arguments
will seem so clearly unanswerable that future generations will wonder why we squandered our funds in helping those who did not need
help. At present, however, Social Security and dozens of other lesser
programs are invariably discussed in terms of rights, not of needs.
The problem of cost, however, cannot be evaded simply by reiterating
the worthiness of the beneficiaries. Nor, more broadly, can platitudi-
nous declarations on social justice obscure the fundamentally political question that must be confronted: in a society with many
claimants jostling for the public purse, how much shall be allocated to
the elderly and on what conditions and for what purposes?

A second approach that is being discussed is the adoption of
policies that permit the aged to make better use of the resources they
possess. Seventy percent of the aged own their own homes—80 percent of these mortgage-free—and this has led to proposals to tap this
vast source of equity. A so-called "reverse mortgage," for example,
would allow the elderly homeowner to borrow against his house, with
the loan repayable upon his death or the sale of the house. Another
scheme would allow elderly homeowners to defer all property taxes
indefinitely. In return, the state would take a lien on the house in the
amount of the deferred taxes plus interest and the heirs would pay
the tax. A third plan entails an elderly person's transfer of his or her
house to a nonprofit agency in return for a monthly check plus free
rent, maintenance, insurance, and tax payments as long as the elder
occupies the house. Upon his death, the house is sold and the equity
applied to finance the program. Variations of these plans have recently been introduced in a half-dozen states, and the federal government has given federally chartered savings and loan associations

permission to issue reverse mortgages since 1979. The great advantage of these plans, proponents assert, is that they permit greater utilization of equity by allowing it to be turned into income. The 1981 White House Conference on Aging supported this approach.

If the home is, typically, the elderly's most important material resource, there also exist the intangible resources of skills, experience, training, and education that could be tapped by having the well elderly postpone their retirement from the workforce. Whereas, in 1950, about 90 percent of men aged 54 to 65 indicated that they planned to retire by age 65, in 1978 the percentage had fallen to 74 and today the figure is said to be even lower.[20] Inflationary pressures that have eroded the value of pensions, savings, and annuities, a 1979 federal law that set the age of mandatory retirement at 70 for most workers, healthier elders, and changing corporate attitudes, have all helped to bring this change about.

Statutory obstacles, however, remain, such as the Social Security penalty for earning over $3,720 (under 65) or $5,000 (age 65 to 71) per year. If this penalty were abolished, it has been suggested,[21] it would encourage a sizable number of the elderly to be more self-supporting. And by taking care of themselves financially, they would enhance their own self-esteem and their public image, as well as reducing the burden on the taxpayer.[22] In the process, of course, Social Security would be made more an annuity than an income replacement system, and yet proponents would observe that Social Security benefits even now replace on the average only 42 percent of preretirement income, anyway. Indeed, what the advocates of the new directions in aging policy seem to be saying is that the American dream of a comfortable, work-free old age for everyone is simply not attainable or perhaps not even desirable, and that prevailing attitudes must change if the realities of the 1980s are to be accommodated.

These plans are not without their drawbacks, and even their most fervent supporters would not describe them as panaceas. Easy talk of the working elderly, for example, runs the risk of ignoring the fact that three-quarters of the men who choose early Social Security retirement are motivated not by the prospect of an idyllic enjoyment of postponed pleasures, but rather by the compulsions of ill health (54 percent) or unemployment (23 percent). Nor is finding work necessarily an achievable goal, given the impact of age discrimination, technological changes, shifting job markets, atrophied job-seeking skills, and simple discouragement.

Nonetheless, targeting government efforts more narrowly at the needy and making greater use of the elderly's own resources are options that demand the attention of interested parties, if only because they illustrate the kind of thinking that now appears on the rise. Some may applaud it and others deplore it, but no one who cares about the place of the aged in America can neglect it for very long.

The difficulty is, however, that the aged and their advocates in the bureaucracy, academia, pressure groups, and the media are so numerous, well-organized, and fearful, that merely questioning the wisdom of current policies is likely to provoke extreme and instantaneous reactions. When the Reagan administration proposed cutting Social Security benefits for those seeking early retirement, for example, it was immediately attacked for "throwing old people to the sharks."[23] Similarly, an effort to eliminate minimum Social Security benefits was termed, "a knife in the heart of the elderly in this country,"[24] though nearly everyone privately conceded that the system was scandalously wasteful. Rhetoric this vivid and damning is not typical of American politics, but it certainly typified discussion of the Reagan proposals. Shortly thereafter, a Gallup poll disclosed that the President's public standing had dropped markedly, partly as a result of his Social Security plan. In addition, a Harris survey found an overwhelming majority of Americans viewing him as unfair to the elderly, and leading Democrats let it be known that they would seek to make Social Security a major issue in the next campaign. Meanwhile, though, near the peak of his popularity, President Reagan saw his Social Security measures rejected by a Senate controlled by his own party by a vote of 96 to 0. A subsequent all-out effort to control a White House Conference on Aging met with only limited success. It would be difficult for even the most obtuse politician to miss the lesson that tinkering with America's aging policies would inflame tens of millions of recipients and hundreds of thousands of private and public employees dependent upon them. A more perilous political undertaking would be difficult to imagine. It is hardly surprising, then, that a chastened Reagan sought to silence the issue during the 1982 elections by appointing a bipartisan task force to engage in yet another study of the problem.

It is surely naive to expect a broad consensus to revise aging programs in an atmosphere full of philosophical calm and free of controversy and venom. Indeed, given the effect of such programs upon the lives of a large portion of society, nothing less than a full and vigorous debate would seem appropriate. At the same time, however, debate can hardly proceed in a context of hysteria, in which name-calling and prophecies of calamity treat rationality like an intruder.

The programs are political—that is, they pivot on who gets what, when, and how—and their future should be determined by the political process. But it should not be too much to hope that the profound and complex issues they represent can call upon the nation's best political instincts, though this is hardly what we have witnessed so far.

Notes

[1] In addition, tax expenditures benefiting only the elderly totalled $9.9 billion in 1980.

[2] "Note: Discrimination Against the Elderly: A Perspective on the Problem," *Suffolk Law Review* 7 (1973):918.

[3] Louis Harris, "Remarks at a Congressional Briefing, November 18, 1981," *Congressional Record* (November 18, 1981), pp. S13673 (daily ed.).

[4] United States House of Representatives, Select Committee on Aging, *Retirement, The Broken Promise* (Washington: Government Printing Office, 1981).

[5] Morton Paglin, "Poverty in the United States: A Reevaluation," *Policy Review,* Vol. 7 (1979):7.

[6] The elderly's homes tend to be older than the average home—but not significantly inferior to it—and are less costly to maintain and repair. R. J. Struyk, *The Housing Situation of Elderly Americans* (Washington: Urban Institute, 1976); U.S. Department of Commerce, Bureau of the Census, *Residential Alterations and Repair: Expenditures on Residential Additions, Alterations, Maintenance, and Replacement, Construction Reports C50-74 Q1 and Q2* (Washington: Government Printing Office, 1974). In fact, 96 percent of aged homeowners profess satisfaction with their housing, and 93 percent say that they have no desire to leave their homes, even for condominiums offering more amenities and no structural defects. Alvin Rabushka and B. Jacobs, *Old Folks at Home* (New York: Free Press, 1980).

[7] Thomas Halper, "The Double-Edged Sword: Paternalism as a Policy in the Problems of Aging," *Milbank Memorial Fund Quarterly* 58 (1980):489–90.

[8] Cf., J. A. M. Gray, "Do We Care Too Much For Our Elders?" *Lancet,* June 14, 1980, pp. 1289–91.

[9] Arthur N. Schwartz, "An Observer: On Self-Esteem as the Linchpin of Quality of Life for the Aged," *Gerontologist* 15 (1975):470.

[10] L. H. Getze, "What the Aging Network Can Do For You," *Modern Maturity,* March-April, 1981, p. 33.

[11] "Editorial: Social Security Can Be Trimmed," *New York Times,* March 13, 1981, p. A30, col. 1; Barbara R. Bergman, "Relax, Social Security Is

Doing Its Job," *New York Times,* November 15, 1981, III, p. 3, col. 1; Eli Ginzberg, "The Social Security System," *Scientific American* 246 (January, 1982):57.

[12]Edward Cowan, "Divided U.S. Advisory Panel Urges Changes in Social Security System," *New York Times,* March 13, 1981, p. A15, col. 5; "Editorial: Time for Surgery on Social Security," *New York Times,* May 10, 1981, p. 18, col. 1; Warren Weaver, Jr., "Cost-Of-Living Raises a Target as Congress Examines Social Security," *New York Times,* July 6, 1981, p. A10, col. 3.

[13]"Editorial: Saving Social Security from Itself," *New York Times,* January 4, 1979, p. A18, col. 1.

[14]Robert M. Ball, *Social Security: Today and Tomorrow* (New York: Columbia University Press, 1978).

[15]So have such long-time defenders of the aged as Senator Lawton Chiles (D-Fla.) and labor economist Eli Ginzberg. See Lawton Chiles, "Address before the White House Conference on Aging," *Congressional Record* (December 2, 1981), pp. S14309–10 and Ginzberg, *loc. cit.*

[16]Cruikshank, quoted in Steven V. Roberts, "Growing U.S. Expenditures for the Aged Cause Concern Among Policymakers," *New York Times,* December 27, 1978, p. B8, col. 1.

[17]Robert B. Hudson, "The 'Graying' of the Federal Budget and Its Consequences for Old-age Policy," *Gerontologist* 18 (1978):439.

[18]Worker-beneficiary ratios have dropped from 50:1 in 1945 to 3.1:1 in 1982, and a further decline to 2.1:1 by 2015 is widely expected. Such distant projections, however, may ignore significant intermediary changes, such as increasing levels of working elderly, gains in labor productivity, or alterations in fertility patterns or immigration policies. It is probably wiser, therefore, to view the future with concern, rather than alarm.

[19]This, of course, raises the question of the application of a means test to Social Security itself. While few propose such a change publicly, their argument clearly is that the system must be viewed as generational transfer payments that threaten to become so expensive that they must be confined to cases of demonstrable need. Others reply that Social Security benefits represent a form of deferred earnings and, insofar as different generations are involved, derive from a contractual obligation between generations that must be respected; even to discuss altering the system, in this view, should be discouraged as inducing fear and anxiety among those no longer well-positioned to cope with such changes. Since the average Social Security recipient receives several times the funds he or she contributed—the average unmarried male worker who retired in 1979 after having earned wages at the maximum level will receive five times as much benefits as contributions, for example, and the average recipient with a dependent spouse who retired in 1979 after having earned wages at the minimum level will receive thirteen times as much benefits as contributions (Ginzberg, *op. cit.* p. 52)—the deferred earnings argument is difficult to take seriously.

[20]E. M. Fowler, "The Trend to Later Retirement," *New York Times,* February 25, 1981, p. D13, col. 1.

[21]M. R. Colberg, *The Social Security Retirement Test,* Washington: American Enterprise Institute for Public Policy Research, 1978; President's Commission on Pension Policy, *Interim Report,* Washington: Government Printing Office, 1980.

[22]Of course, this would also discourage the elderly from retiring and opening up jobs for younger workers with families to support; but this may be only a short-run problem, for demographers project that by 2010 there will be only three younger job seekers for every four older workers—not even the replacement rate.

[23]Ossofsky, quoted in Warren Weaver, Jr., "Coalition Plans Drive Against Move to Trim Social Security Benefits," *New York Times,* May 14, 1981, p. B15, col. 1.

[24]Pryor, quoted in "Parties in Senate Exchange Barbs on Aid to Aged," *New York Times,* March 31, 1981, p. A6, col. 1.

2

Is Aging a Disease?

ARTHUR L. CAPLAN

Normality, Naturalness, and Disease

The belief that aging is a normal and natural part of human existence is commonplace in the practice of medicine. For example, no mention is made in most textbooks in the areas of medicine and pathology of aging as abnormal, unnatural, or indicative of disease. It is true that such texts often contain a chapter or two on the related subject of diseases commonly associated with aging or found in the elderly. But it is these diseases frequently encountered in the elderly—such as pneumonia, cancer, or atherosclerosis—rather than the aging process itself, that serve as the focus of description and analysis.

Why should this situation exist? What is so different about the physiological changes and deteriorations of the aging process that these events are considered to be unremarkable natural processes, while apparently similar processes in a young person are deemed to be diseases constituting health crises of the first order? Surely it cannot simply be the life-threatening aspects of diseases, like cancer or atherosclerosis, that distinguish them from aging. For while it may be true that hardly anyone manages to avoid contracting a terminal disease at some point in life, aging itself produces the same ultimate consequence as these diseases. Nor can it be the familiarity

Portions of this paper were read at the University of Western Ontario and New York University. I am grateful for the comments I received at these schools and for the suggestions of the members of the Project on Ethics and Values of Columbia University.

and universality of aging that inure medical science to its unnatural aspects. Malignant neoplasms, viral infections, and hypertension are all ubiquitous phenomena. Yet medicine maintains a stance toward these physical processes that is radically different from that which it holds toward the so-called "natural" changes that occur during aging.

What seems to differentiate aging from other processes or states traditionally classified as diseases is the fact that aging is perceived as a natural or normal process. Medicine has traditionally viewed its role as that of ameliorating or combating the abnormal, either through therapeutic interventions or preventive, prophylactic regimens. The natural and the normal, while not outside the sphere of medicine, are concepts that play key roles in licensing the intervention of the medical practitioner. For it is in response to or in anticipation of abnormality that physicians' activities are legitimated. As E. A. Murphy, among many other clinicians, has noted, "The clinician has tended to regard disease as that state in which the limits of the normal have been transgressed."[1] Naturalness and normality have, historically, been used as baselines to determine the presence of disease and the necessity of medical activity.

In light of the powerful belief that the abnormal and unnatural are indicative of medicine's range of interest, it is easy to see why many biological processes are not thought to be the proper subject of medical intervention or therapy. Puberty, growth, and maturation *as processes in themselves* all appear to stand outside the sphere of medical concern since they are normal and natural occurrences among human beings. Similarly, it seems odd to think of sexuality or fertilization as possible disease states precisely because these states are commonly thought to be natural and normal components of the human condition.

Nonetheless, it is true that certain biological processes, such as conception, pregnancy, and fertility, have been the subject in recent years of heated debates as to their standing as possible disease states. The notions that it is natural and normal for only men and women to have sexual intercourse or for women to undergo menopause have been challenged in many quarters. The question arises as to whether the process of aging in and of itself can be classified as abnormal and unnatural in a way that will open the door for the reclassification of aging as a disease process and, thus, a proper subject of medical attention, concern, and control.

Aging and Medical Intervention

The status of aging and dying as natural processes looms especially large in current discussions about the "right to die" and "death with dignity." Often those who debate the degree to which the medical profession should intervene in the process of dying disagree about the naturalness of the phenomena of aging and dying. If the alleged right to die is to be built on a conception of the naturalness of aging and dying, then the conceptual status of these terms vis-à-vis "naturalness" must be thoroughly examined. The question of the naturalness of aging, senescence, and death must not be permitted to become lost in complex debates concerning the rights and obligations of patients and health professionals.

As noted earlier, the perception of biological events or processes as natural or unnatural is frequently decisive in determining whether physicians treat certain states or processes as diseases.[2] One need only think of the controversies that swirl around allegations concerning the biological naturalness of homosexuality or schizophrenia to see that this is so. This claim is further borne out by an argument that is frequently made by older physicians to new medical students. Medical students often find it difficult to interact with or examine elderly patients. They may feel powerless when confronted with the seemingly irreversible debilities of old age. To overcome this reluctance, older physicians are likely to point out that aging is a process that happens to everyone, even young medical students. Aging is simply part of the human condition; it should hold no terror for a young doctor. Students are told that aging is natural and that, while there may be nothing they can do to alter the inevitable course of this process, they must learn to help patients cope with their aging as best they can. It is as if teaching physicians feel obligated to label the obviously debilitative and disease-like states of old age as natural in order to discourage the students' inclination to treat the elderly as sick or diseased.

What is Aging?

Why do we think of aging as a natural process? The reason that comes immediately to mind is that aging is a common and normal process. It occurs with a statistical frequency of one hundred percent. Inevitably and uniformly bones become brittle, vision dims, joints stiffen, and muscles lose their tone. The obvious question that arises is whether commonality, familiarity, and inevitability are sufficient conditions for describing certain biological states as natural. To answer this question, it is necessary first to draw a distinction between aging and chronological age.

In a trivial sense, given the existence of a chronological device, all bodies that exist can be said to age relative to the measurements provided by that device. But since physicians have little practical interest in making philosophical statements about the time-bound nature of existence, or empirical claims about the relativity of space and time, it is evident that they do not have this chronological sense in mind in speaking about the familiarity and inevitability of aging.

In speaking of aging, physicians are interested in a particular set of biological changes that occur with respect to time. These changes occur at a variety of levels in human beings. At the molecular level, extensive research has shown substantial changes in enzyme activity among the elderly. At the cellular level, increase in age is correlated with increases in the length of the cell cycle during mitosis. At the level of organs and tissues, aging is correlated with deterioration in various joints, a decline in body potassium, wrinkled skin, thickening of the lens of the eye, a decline in immune function, and a decline in lung capacity.

There is a distinct set of psychological changes that constitute the aging process as well. For example, long-term memory tends to decline with age. Perceptual abilities, such as visual acuity, depth perception, color discrimination, taste sensitivity, and pitch discrimination tend to decline as one becomes older. There are general declines in many intellectual abilities, particularly those involving speed of response in nonverbal, manipulative skills.

These types of cellular, organic, and psychological changes constitute the aging process. They do not occur at the same rate in all persons and do not proceed at the same rate within any particular individual. It is this set of biological and psychological changes[3]— not the mere passage of time—that constitutes the phenomenon of aging.

Studies on animals show that similar patterns of change can be found occurring at different rates in a wide variety of mammals. It is also interesting to note that the genetic disease, progeria, which afflicts young children, presents many of the same biological and psychological changes associated with the aging process. Variations among normal human beings in the degree to which the signs of aging occur, and the fact that some young humans can be afflicted with the signs of aging, reveal that age and aging must be understood as distinct, although related, phenomena.

Naturalness, Design, and Function

While it is true that aging occurs at different rates in different people, such changes are universal and eventually inevitable. Universality and inevitability do not, however, seem to be sufficient conditions for referring to a process as natural. Coronary atherosclerosis, neoplasms, high blood pressure, sore throats, colds, tooth decay, and depression are all nearly universal in their distribution, and are seemingly inevitable phenomena. Yet it seems awkward to call these phenomena natural processes or states. The inevitability of infection by microorganisms among all humans does not cause the physician to dismiss these infections as natural occurrences of no particular medical interest. The physician may not intervene, nor even attempt to prevent such diseases, but such behavior is a result of a decision concerning an unnatural disease, not a natural process.

If universality and inevitability are not adequate criteria for defining naturalness, are any other criteria available by which naturalness can be assessed and used to drive a wedge between aging and disease? There is another sense of "natural"[4] that may prove helpful in trying to understand why physicians are reluctant to label aging a disease, preferring to think of it as a natural process.

This sense of naturalness is rooted in the notions of design, purpose, and function. Axes are designed to serve as tools for cutting trees. Scalpels are meant to be used in cutting human tissue. It would seem most unnatural to use axes for surgery and scalpels for lumberjacking. In some sense, although a skillful surgeon might, in fact, be able to perform surgery with an axe, it would be unnatural to do so. Similarly, many bodily organs—the liver, spleen, blood vessels, kidneys, and many glands—can perform a variety of functions. They can even compensate for the functions of organic tissues that are damaged. But these are not the purposes or functions they were "designed" to perform. While the arteries of many organisms are capable of constricting to maintain blood pressure and reduce the flow of blood during hemorrhage-induced shock, one essential function of the arteries is not to constrict in response to such circumstances. The presence of vasoconstriction in arteries is, in fact, an unnatural state that signals the physician that something has gone seriously awry in the body. It may be that much of our willingness to accept aging as a natural process is dependent upon some sense of "natural" function.

Two answers are commonly given to the question: What is the function of aging? The first is a theological explanation. God, in punishment for the sins of our ancestors in the (proverbial) garden of Eden, caused humans to age and die. On this view, people age because the Creator saw fit to design them that way for retribution or punishment. Aging serves as a reminder of our moral fallibility and weakness.

The second view, which is particularly widespread in scientific circles, is that the purpose or function of aging is to clear away the old to make way for the new for evolutionary reasons. This theory was first advanced by the German cytologist and evolutionary biologist August Weismann at the turn of the century.[5] Weismann argued that aging and debilitation must be viewed as adaptational responses on the part of organisms to allow for new mutational and adaptive responses to fluctuating environments. Aging benefits the population by removing the superannuated to make room for the young. The function of aging is to ensure the death of organisms to allow evolutionary change and new adaptation to occur.

In both of these views aging has an intended purpose or function. And it is from this quasi-Aristotelian attribution of a design that the "naturalness" of aging is often thought to arise.

The Concept of Biological Function

Rooting the source of the naturalness of biological processes in ideas of function or purpose has its drawbacks, the primary one being that philosophers have by no means reached anything even vaguely resembling a consensus about the meaning of such terms as "function" or "purpose."

Fortunately, it is possible to avoid becoming bogged down in an analysis of functional or purposive statements in analyzing the function of aging. The only distinction required for understanding the function of aging is that between the aim of explaining the existence of a particular state, organ, or process, and that of explaining how a state, organ, or process works in a particular system or organism. Functional or purposive statements are sometimes used to explain the existence of a trait or process, historically. At other times, such statements are used mechanistically to explain how something works or operates. If we ask what is the function, or role, or purpose of the spleen in the human body, the question can be interpreted in two ways: How does the spleen work—what does it do in the body? Or, why does the spleen exist in its present state in the human body—what is the historical story that explains why persons have spleens?[6]

It is this latter sense of function, the historical sense, that is relevant to the determination of the naturalness or unnaturalness of aging as a biological process. For while there is no shortage of theories purporting to explain how aging works or functions, these theories are not relevant to the historically motivated question about the function of aging. The determination of the naturalness of aging, if it is to be rooted in biology, will depend not on how the process of aging actually operates, but rather on the explanation one gives for the existence or presence of aging in humans.[7]

Does Aging Have a Function?

Two purported explanations—one theological, one scientific—of the function or purpose of aging have been given. Both are flawed. While the theological explanation of aging may carry great weight for numerous individuals, it will simply not do as a scientific explanation of why aging occurs in humans. Medical professionals may have to cope with their patients' advocacy of this explanation and their own religious feelings on the subject. But, from a scientific perspective, it will hardly do to claim that aging, as a result of God's vindictiveness, is a natural biological process, and hence not a disease worthy of treatment.

More surprisingly, the scientific explanation of aging as serving an evolutionary role or purpose is also inadequate. It is simply not true that aging exists to serve any sort of evolutionary purpose or function. The claim that aging exists or occurs in individuals because it has a wider role or function in the evolutionary scheme of things rests on faulty evolutionary analysis. The analysis incorrectly assumes that it is possible for biological processes to exist that directly benefit or advance the evolutionary success of a species or population.

Evolutionary selection rarely acts to advance the prospects of an entire species or population. Selection acts on individual organisms and their phenotypic traits and properties. Some traits or properties confer advantages in certain environments on the organisms that possess them and this fact increases the likelihood that the genes responsible for producing these traits will be passed on to future organisms.

Given that selective forces act on individuals and their geno-
types and not species, it makes no sense to speak of aging as serving
an evolutionary function or purpose to benefit the species. How then
do evolutionary biologists explain the existence of aging?[8] Briefly,
the explanation is that features, traits, or properties in individual
organisms will be selected for if they confer a relative reproductive
advantage on the individual or his or her close kin. Any variation
that increases inclusive reproductive fitness has a very high probability of being selected and maintained in the gene pool of a species.
Selection, however, cannot look ahead to foresee the possible consequences of favoring certain traits at a given time; the environment
selects for those traits and features that give an immediate return.
An increased metabolic rate, for example, may prove advantageous
early in life in that it may provide more energy for seeking mates and
avoiding predators; it may also result in early deterioration of the
organism due to an increased accumulation of toxic wastes in the
body of an individual thus endowed. Natural selection cannot foresee
such delayed debilitating consequences.

Aging exists, then, as a consequence of a lack of evolutionary
foresight; it is simply a by-product of selective forces which increase
the chances of reproductive success in the life of an organism. Senescence has no function; it is simply the inadvertent subversion of
organic function, later in life, in favor of maximizing reproductive
advantage, early in life.

The common belief that aging serves a function or purpose is
based on a misapprehension of evolutionary processes. It would
further seem that the common belief that aging is a natural process,
as a consequence of the function or purpose it serves in the life of the
species, is also mistaken. Consequently, unless it is possible to moti-
vate the description on other grounds, it would seem that aging
cannot be understood as a natural process. And if that is true, and if it
is actually the case that what goes on during the aging process closely
parallels the changes that occur during paradigmatic examples of
disease,[9] then it would be unreasonable not to consider aging as a
disease.

Theories of Aging and the Concept of Disease

A consideration of the changes that constitute aging in human beings
reinforces the similarities existing between aging and other clear-cut
examples of somatic diseases. There is a set of external manifesta-

tions or symptoms: greying hair, increased susceptibility to infection, wrinkling skin, loss of muscular tone, and, frequently, loss of some mental ability. These manifestations seem to be causally linked to a series of internal cellular and subcellular changes. The presence of symptoms and an underlying etiology closely parallel the standard paradigmatic examples of disease. If the analogy is pushed a bit further, the case for considering aging a disease appears to become even stronger.

There are many theories as to what causes changes, at the cellular and subcellular level, that produce the signs and symptoms associated with aging.[10] One view argues that aging is caused by an increase in the number of cross-linkages that exist in protein and nucleic acid molecules. Cross-linkages lower the biochemical efficiency and dependability of certain macromolecules involved in metabolism and other chemical reactions. Free radical by-products of metabolism are thought to accumulate in cells, thus allowing for an increase in available linkage sites for replicating nucleic acid strands and activating histone elements. This sort of cross-linkage is thought to be particularly important in the aging of collagen, the substance responsible for most of the overt symptoms we commonly associate with aging, such as wrinkled skin and loss of muscular flexibility.

Another view holds that aging results from an accumulation of genetic mutations in the chromosomes of cells in the body. The idea underlying this theory is that chromosomes are exposed over time to a steady stream of radiation and other mutagenic agents. The accumulation of mutational hits on the genes lying on the chromosomes results in the progressive inactivation of these genes. The evidence of a higher incidence of chromosomal breaks and aberrations in the aged is consistent with this mutational theory of aging.

Along with the cross-linkage and mutational theories, there is one other important hypothesis concerning the causes of aging. The auto-immune theory holds that, as time passes and the chromosomes of cells in the human body accumulate more mutations, certain key tissues begin to synthesize antibodies that can no longer distinguish between self and foreign material. Thus, a number of auto-immune reactions occur in the body as the immunological system begins to turn against the individual it was "designed" to protect. Certain types of arthritis and pernicious anemia are examples of debilities resulting from the malfunction of the immunological system. While this theory is closely allied to the mutation theory, the auto-immune view of aging holds that accumulated mutations do not simply result in deterioration of cellular activity but, rather, produce lethal cellular end products that consume and destroy healthy tissue.

It would be rash to hold that any of the three hypotheses cited— the cross-linkage, mutational, or auto-immune hypotheses—will, in the end, turn out to be *the* correct explanation of aging. All three views are, in fact, closely related in that cross-linkages can result from periodic exposure to mutagenic agents and can, in turn, produce genetic aberrations which eventuate in cellular dysfunction or even auto-immune reactions. What is important, however, is not whether *one* of these theories is in fact *the* correct theory of aging, but that all of the current plausible theories postulate mechanisms that are closely analogous to those mechanisms cited by clinicians when describing other disease processes in the body.

The concept of disease is, without doubt, a slippery and evasive notion in medicine.[11] Once one moves away from what can be termed "paradigmatic" examples of disease, such as tuberculosis and diphtheria, toward more nebulous examples, such as acne or jittery nerves, it becomes difficult to say exactly what are the criteria requisite for labeling a condition a somatic disease. However, even though it is notoriously difficult to concoct a set of necessary and sufficient conditions for employing the term "organic disease," it is possible to cite a list of general criteria that seem relevant in attempting to decide whether a bodily state or process is appropriately labeled a disease.

One criterion is that the state or process produces discomfort or suffering. A second is that the process or state can be traced back to a specific cause, event, or circumstance. A third is that there is a set of clear-cut structural changes, both macroscopic and microscopic, that follow in a uniform, sequential manner subsequent to the initial precipitating or causal event. A fourth is that there is a set of clinical symptoms or manifestations (headache, pain in the chest, rapid pulse, shortness of breath) commonly associated with the observed physiological alterations in structure. Finally,[12] there is usually some sort of functional impairment in the abilities, behavior, or activity of a person thought to be diseased. Not all diseases will satisfy all or any of these criteria. One need only consider the arguments surrounding the proper classification of astigmatism, alcoholism, drug addiction, gambling, and hyperactivity to realize the limited resolving power of these criteria. Nevertheless, advocates of all persuasions regarding controversial states and processes commonly resort to considerations of causation, clinical manifestations, etiology, functional impairment, and suffering in arguing the merits of their various views concerning the disease status of controversial cases.

With respect to the conceptual ambiguity surrounding the notion of disease, it is important to remember that medicine is by no means unique in being saddled with what might be termed "fuzzy-edged" concepts. One need only consider the status of terms such as "species," "adaptation," and "mutation" in biology, or "stimulus," "behavior," or "instinct" in psychology to realize that medicine is not alone in the ambiguity of its key terms. It is also true that, just as the biologist is able to use biological theory to aid in the determination of relevant criteria and their fulfillment for a concept, the physician—as many writers have noted—is able to use his or her knowledge of the structure, design, and function of the body to decide upon relevant criteria for the determination of disease.

If one accepts the relevance of the five suggested criteria, then aging, as a biological process, is seen to possess all the key properties of a disease. Unlike alcoholism or nervousness, aging possesses a definitive group of clinical manifestations or symptoms; a clear-cut etiology of structural changes at both the macroscopic and microscopic levels; a significant measure of impairment, discomfort, and suffering; and, if we are willing to grant the same tolerance to current theories of aging as we grant to theories in other domains of medicine, an explicit set of precipitating factors. Aging has all the relevant markings of a disease process. And if my earlier argument is sound, even if an additional criterion of unnaturalness is added to these five, aging would still meet all the requirements thought relevant to the classification of a process or state as indicative of disease.

Some Ethical Arguments Against Treating Aging as a Disease

What consequences hinge on the decision to refer to a process or state such as aging by the word "disease" rather than by some other term? Obviously, a great deal. Medical attention, medical support, medical treatment, and medical research are devoted to the treatment, care, amelioration, and prevention of disease. While it is possible to view the activation of this vast professional machine either as a positive good or as a serious evil, an array of implications surrounds the decision of the medical profession to consider a phenomenon worthy of its attention. Some groups have actively proselytized for the acceptance of certain conditions, such as alcoholism or gambling, as diseases. Other groups have worked to remove the label of disease from behavior such as homosexuality, masturbation, and schizophrenia. A number of motives and concerns underlie these arguments. The question is, what kinds of value considerations should be considered relevant to the determination of whether a particular state, process, or condition is a disease?

I do not propose to try to answer the difficult question of what are the relevant nonorganic criteria affecting the choice of the disease label. Rather, I want to consider three specific arguments that might be raised against calling aging a disease—a classification that, of necessity, keeps the aged in touch with the medical profession.

The first counterargument is that the decision to call aging a disease would be pointless, since doctors cannot at present intervene to treat or cure aging. This argument does not stand up to critical scrutiny. There are many diseases in existence today for which no cure is known, but no one proposes that these disorders are any less diseases as a consequence. Furthermore, the emphasis on treatment and cure implicit in this argument ignores the equally vital components of medical care involving understanding, education, and research. The interest of the patient and profession in the healing function of medicine might make it difficult for physicians to accept aging as a disease, but the difficulty in achieving such acceptance does not provide a reason for rejecting the view.

The second argument is that to call aging a disease would involve the stigmatization of a large segment of the population; to view the aged as sick or diseased would only increase the burdens already borne by this much abused segment of society. The problem with this argument is that it tends to blur public perceptions of disease in general with the particular problem of seeing aging as a disease and the ensuing undesirable connotations. To deny that aging is a disease may simply be an easy way to avoid the more difficult problem of educating the medical profession and the lay public toward a better understanding of the threatening and nonthreatening aspects of disease. Contagiousness, death, disability, and neglect may be the real objects of concern in stigmatizing disease, not disease in itself.

Finally, it might be claimed that there would be a tremendous social and economic cost to calling aging a disease. The claim is perhaps the most unconvincing of the three that I have offered. One factor especially relevant to the determination or diagnosis of disease would seem to be that the physician confine his or her concerns to the physical and mental state of the individual patient; social and economic considerations would appear to be quite out of place. Genetic and psychological diseases place a large burden on society; dialysis machines and tomography units are enormously expensive. But these facts do not in any way change the disease status of mongolism, schizophrenia, kidney failure, or cancer. It may be the case that the government might decide not to spend one cent on research into aging or the treatment of aging. But such a decision should be consequent on, not prior to, a diagnosis of disease. This argument simply confounds the value questions relevant to a decision as to whether something is a disease with value questions relevant to deciding what to do about something after it has been decided that it is a disease.

I have suggested a number of possible value issues and social problems that may enter into the decision of the medical profession to label a state or process a disease.[13] I have also suggested that none of these issues and problems would seem to rule out a consideration of aging as a disease. The determination of disease status and the question of how physicians and society should react to disease are distinct issues. Considerations of the latter variety ought not to be allowed to color our decisions about what does and what does not constitute a disease.

Most persons in our society would be loath to see aging classified and treated as a disease. Much of the resistance to such a classification derives from the view that aging is a natural process and that, like other natural processes, it ought not, in itself, be the subject of medical intervention and therapeutic control. I have tried to show that much of the reasoning that tacitly underlies the categorization of aging as a natural or normal process rests on faulty biological analysis. Aging is not the goal or aim of the evolutionary process. Rather it is an accidental by-product of that process. Accordingly, it is incorrect to root a belief in the naturalness of aging in some sort of perceived biological design or purpose since aging serves no such end. It may be that good arguments can be adduced for excluding aging from the purview of medicine. However, if such arguments can be made, they must draw on considerations other than that of the naturalness of aging.[14] Given the parallels that exist between aging and other paradigmatic cases of disease, there would appear to be no reason not to classify aging as a disease.

Notes

[1] E. A. Murphy, *The Logic of Medicine* (Baltimore: Johns Hopkins University Press, 1976), p. 122. See also E. A. Murphy, "A Scientific Viewpoint on Normalcy," *Perspectives in Biology and Medicine*; and G. B. Risse, "Health and Disease: History of the Concepts," in *Encyclopedia of Bioethics*, W. T. Reich, ed. (New York: The Free Press, 1978), pp. 579–585.

[2] S. Goldberg, "What is 'Normal'?: Logical Aspects of the Question of Homosexual Behavior," *Psychiatry* 38 (1975):227–242; Charles Socarites, "Homosexuality and Medicine," *Journal of the American Medical Association* 212 (1970):1199–1202; and I. Illich, "The Political Uses of Natural Death," *Hastings Center Studies* 2 (1974): 3–20.

[3] See E. Palmore, "United States of America" in E. Palmore (ed.), *International Handbook on Aging* (Westport, CN: Greenwood Press, 1980), pp. 434–454, for further discussion of the nature of aging.

[4] See D. B. Hausman, Cf., "What Is Natural?," *Perspectives in Biology and Medicine* 19 (1975):92–101, for an illuminating discussion of the concept.

[5] A. Weismann, *Essays Upon Heredity and Kindred Biological Problems*, 2d ed. (Oxford: Clarendon Press, 1891).

[6] For a sample of the extant explications of the concept of function, see L. Wright, "Functions," *Philosophical Review* 82 (1973):139–168; R. Cummins, "Functional Analysis," *Journal of Philosophy* 72 (1975): 741–765; and M. A. Boden, *Purposive Explanation in Psychology*, Cambridge, Mass., Harvard (1972). See also E. Nagel, *Teleology Revisited*, New York: Columbia, (1979).

[7] Further discussion of the distinction between explaining the operation of a trait or feature and explaining the origin and presence of a trait or feature can be found in A. L. Caplan, "Evolution, Ethics and the Milk of Human Kindness," *Hastings Center Report* 6:2 (1976), pp. 20–26.

[8] G. C. Williams, *Adaptation and Natural Selection* (Princeton: Princeton University Press, 1966); and M. T. Ghiselin, *The Economy of Nature and the Evolution of Sex* (Berkeley: University of California Press, 1974).

[9] For an interesting attempt to analyze the concepts of illness and disease, see C. Boorse, "On the Distinction Between Illness and Disease," *Philosophy and Public Affairs* 5:1 (1975), pp. 49–68.

[10] A. Comfort, "Biological Theories of Aging," *Human Development* 13 (1970): 127–39; L. Hayflick, "The Biology of Human Aging," *American Journal of Medical Sciences* 265:6 (1973), pp. 433–45; A. Comfort, *Aging: The Biology of Senescence* (New York: Holt, Rinehart and Winston, 1964).

[11] R. M. Veatch, "The Medical Model: Its Nature and Problems," *Hastings Center Studies* 1:3 (1973), pp. 59–76.

[12] Boorse, "On the Distinction Between Illness and Disease."

[13] The role played by values in explicating the concepts of health and disease

is notoriously controversial. See, for example, J. Margolis, "The Concept of Disease," *Journal of Medicine and Philosophy* 1 (1976):238–255. I do not wish to enter this debate here. Rather, I simply am making the point that if aging is to avoid the label of disease, it must be on valuational grounds alone.

[14]Certainly arguments can be made against ageism regardless of the disease status of aging. See D. H. Fischer, "Putting Our Heads to the 'Problem' of Old Age," in R. Gross, B. Gross, and S. Seidman (eds.), *The New Old: Struggling For Decent Aging* (Garden City, NY: Anchor, 1978), pp. 58–63.

3

Philosophical Reflections on the "Biology of Aging"

STUART F. SPICKER

A hen is only an egg's way of making another egg.
Samuel Butler, *Life and Habit* (1877)

Introduction: The Devaluation of Aging and the Aged

Aside from the poets' eulogies to old age, their bitter odes to its decrepitude, and biogerontologists' descriptions of the cellular deterioration of the aging human body, what can one find in the intellectual literature of our Western heritage that bypasses the culs-de-sac of sentimentality, pseudo-clinical compassion, and fashionable nods to the destructive biases against the aged members of the human commonwealth? The honest answer—"virtually nothing."

Now is it for a philosopher, any more than anyone else, to add his or her voice in support of the disenfranchised, many of whom are aged and poor? And if so, is there a contribution for philosophy and the humanities to make which goes beyond clarifying concepts under the rubrics of "aging" and "the aged"? Can philosophy do more than merely distinguish between 1) chronological age, 2) biological age,

I wish to acknowledge my appreciation to Professor Marvin L. Tanzer of the Department of Biochemistry, School of Medicine, University of Connecticut. Thanks to Professor Tanzer's guidance, I was able to locate the essential biological literature bearing on this chapter, especially the unpublished papers delivered at the Biological Mechanisms in Aging Conference, held June 23–25, 1980, and sponsored by the National Institute on Aging, Bethesda, Maryland. I also wish to thank Susan Corrente, Sally Gadow, Richard Ratzan, and Kathleen Woodward for their extremely helpful suggestions which enabled me to work to improve this essay.

and 3) our experienced, subjective, phenomenological age, the "age" that we feel? Furthermore, when did interest in life span (longevity) along with disease prevention or postponement[1] outrun all interest in senescence, in what the psychologist G. Stanley Hall calls "senectitude, the postclimacteric, old age proper"?[2] Have we, while hypnogogic, imbibed our Darwinian heritage? The fact is, of course, that we are much too Darwinian. We have, that is, quite unreflectively extrapolated conclusions from the fundamental tenets of Darwin's theory of evolution, neglecting in the process to notice that the Darwinian theory necessarily includes a critical value-laden component.

The Influence of Darwinism on the Concept of "Aging" (Senescence)

The appeal to Darwin's theory of natural selection has too frequently led advocates of the aged to accept the thesis that, since the aged members of the species *homo sapiens* have by dint of biological, environmental, social, and cultural factors survived, they are the most "fit" of the species and deserve therefore our admiration, respect, and continued care in their senescent years. But an appeal to Darwin and his revolutionary theory of evolution is, in reality, a futile one when considering the function of the aged. For Darwin's theory begins and ends (one might say) with the notion of reproduction,[3] which is distinct from all earlier theories of generation.[4] It may be of interest briefly to recall the deductive arguments at the core of Darwin's theory. The theory is based on three observations and two deductions:

Observation 1: All organisms tend to multiply in a geometrical fashion. That is, generally speaking offspring are always more numerous than their parents.

Observation 2: Notwithstanding the tendency to increase progressively, the actual number of a given species tends to remain constant over time.

Deduction 1: The existence of individuals and species is the result of a continuous "struggle" for adaptability and competition for survival. That is, since the actual number of young progeny exceeds the number that eventually survive, there must be competition for survival and this includes competition with respect to the events of fertilization and reproduction (especially when sexual reproduction is the means, as is the case for the higher primates).

Observation 3: There is great variation among organisms. That is, not all members of a given species are alike. (The concept of "heritability" is offered as an explanation of variation.)

Deduction 2: Some variations which appear are advantageous for the survival and reproduction of the species; some variations are disadvantageous or unfavorable, and the individuals die or fail to reproduce themselves.

In short, a higher proportion of individuals with favorable variations and traits will survive and reproduce; similarly, a higher proportion of those organisms with unfavorable traits will fail to reproduce. Since only those members of a species capable of producing progeny affect the survival of that species, it follows that only those members of a species capable of reproducing are valued from the standpoint of the theory of natural selection. In fact, one might correctly construe the impact of Darwin's general theory of the mutability of species as serving to disenfranchise further the senescent members of our species, especially the females, since they no longer have the capacity to reproduce (though they need not, of course, forfeit their sexuality). The males, of course, might also be devalued, since they can never bear young. In other words, from the standpoint of Darwinian theory, postmenopausal or senescent females are by definition "evolutionarily irrelevant," and in many instances so too are the males. Making salient the value-laden dimensions of Darwinism, then, we see that members of the species who are incapable of "transmitting progeny," that is, those growing old, are no longer considered relevant, or of much value or interest with regard to the long-term ends of the complex processes of selection, extinction, and survival, which are the *ideés maîtresses* in *The Origin of Species.*

The term "senescence" ("aging") is typically employed by biogerontologists to signal what is for them an essentially deteriorative process.[5] Bernard Strehler cites Alex Comfort: "What is being measured, when we measure it, is a decrease in viability and an increase in vulnerability. Other definitions are possible but they tend to ignore the raison d'être of human and scientific concern with age processes. Senescence shows itself as an increasing probability of death with increasing chronological age."[6] Thus the biological literature on aging reveals such notions as "dermatologic senescence,"[7] "senescent changes in cells,"[8] and "innate or ingrained senescence."[9] Two other biologists define senescence as "the postmaturation decline in survivorship and fecundity that accompanies advancing age."[10] It is clear that the Darwinian heritage is profoundly influential for these scientists. These same authors, in their discussions of *Drosophila melanogaster*, remark that "Mean daily egg lay shows senescent decline, from around 70 eggs per day for the first day of assay to about 30 eggs per day for the last day of assay...."[11] Hence, "observed decline in mean fecundity" and "decrease in early reproductive output" serve to describe the senescence of *Drosophila*. The concept of senescence adapted by biogerontologists, then, is easily appropriated from the Darwinian heritage. Senescence is tightly linked to the failure to reproduce or to be fecund. The influence of Darwinism on the concept of senescence is apparent in the transition from the notion of a species which "transmits progeny" to the notion of cellular replication and reproduction of germ cells, that in August Weismann's view exemplify an unbroken chain of genetic succession extending back to the very first self-reproducing cell.[12]

One need not continue to cite the eminent biogerontologists any further. What is transparent is that their definition of the penultimate phase of human personal life, when applied at the cellular and subcellular levels, fails to convince. Something has gone awry. A subtle, adroit, and almost reflexive linguistic move has seduced us into reducing a term ordinarily descriptive of the personal, post-maturational level and taking it to the cellular and subcellular levels. This is surely an unacceptable move.

Consider the concept of aging or senescent person which lies behind it. Strehler's position is worth underscoring: "In organisms reproducing exclusively by sexual means there appears to be no difficulty in defining individuals—an individual is a collection of cells or organelles functioning in an integrated manner in response to environmental stimuli."[13] One need not dwell on the naive metaphysics suggested here. Suffice it to say that individuals—old persons for example—are not "a collection of cells or organelles" nor is human aging and growing old simply the inability to reproduce, that is, a decrease in the capacity to "transmit progeny." But before we turn to the truly insidious effect which the biological notion of senescence perpetuates, it is necessary to clarify various notions of time which, having remained conflated, only serve to confuse us.

Time, Age, Cells, and Aging Persons

As has been pointed out in a famous passage from St. Augustine's *Confessions,* familiarity with the everyday prevents insight: "What is time? As long as nobody asks me, I know. The moment I want to explain to someone who has asked me, I know not." Yet does not every child learn to tell time? Is not our whole Western life regulated by clock and calendar, timetables and schedules? Does anyone stop to ask what is meant by a day, a week, a year, except perhaps those elderly who suffer from multiple health problems and find themselves all too often with more than enough time on their hands? Even the temporal measurement of events and processes (chronometry) confronts us with the amazing fact that we—living in time—can nevertheless conceive of time; we can scientifically measure biological events and processes, and express the results in terms which biologists, for example, can share. The *chronometry* of cellular and subcellular processes is certainly of great importance to the correctness of inferences drawn by scientists as they attend to these processes. And it is precisely at these levels that one can challenge biologists in terms of their claim that they study *biological mechanisms of aging.* Before continuing let me be perfectly clear: In what follows I do not intend to suggest that the research efforts of many biologists—even and especially those who claim to conduct "research on aging"—is in any way unimportant. That judgment is for biologists to make with regard to one another's specific research efforts, hypotheses, methods, analyses—in short, the adopted standards and norms which scientists have always required of one another.

What I shall argue is that, of the three types of research efforts that are subsumed under the rubric "biology of aging," none qualifies as biological research into human aging. Indeed, my thesis is that biologists are either engaged in research pertinent to 1) human longevity or life span, or 2) the prevention and/or postponement of diseases, many of which presently appear during senescence, or 3) cellular and subcellular processes at the microlevel which are then incoherently extrapolated to macrolevel phenomena, for example, the processes which take place in the cells of the skin are offered as an account of wrinkling, a common external "marker" of aging. Put positively, aging *is* a phenomenon of personal biography, a phenomenon of the social world, and not captured by a linear model of time.

It will soon become evident that many commonly employed terms in the gerontological literature are used equivocally and lead—as they are certain to do—to confusion and incoherence. For instance, consider this excerpt from the "Special Report on Aging, 1980": "In an effort to understand what is meant by the 'aging process,' scientists supported by the NIA [National Institute on Aging] are looking at the changes that take place in animals as they age."[14] In this sentence it is clear that the term "age" is meant to denote the chronological time from birth to death. The passage continues:

> It has long been known that rats whose diets are severely restricted
> during adulthood live longer than those given unlimited access to food.
> But it is not known why this occurs or what relation such diet-induced
> longevity has to *age-related* changes.[15]

Here the author of the *Report* employs the term "longevity," which
refers to the chronological limit of the rat's life span only, but it is
unclear what "age-related" refers to. In all likelihood the term refers
to changes at set points or moments along a linear time dimension as
the rat lives from adulthood to death. The paragraph closes with a
final question: "Do the rats age more slowly or are they less suscepti-
ble to disease?"[16] This question makes clear that the term "age" does
not refer only to chronological (chronometric) time. After all—as
Aristotle already made clear—the interval between minutes or
seconds is *fixed*. It therefore makes no sense at all to speak of "aging
more slowly" or "aging more quickly" when time in the sense of clock
time is being employed. "Age more slowly" or "age more quickly" are
relative notions that can only make sense if, given a linear scale
divided into equal units, (e.g., weeks, months, or years) we plot
against it "ideal" phases. For example, outer markers of age, like the
changes noted in the texture of the skin surface over time, occur
within typical chronological ranges. One might say that wrinkling
begins to appear between chronological ages 40 and 50. It is this
"marker" that, compared to the objective chronometric line, may be
said to appear more slowly or more rapidly in different persons.

In fairness to the biologist, it should be noted that they often
distinguish chronological age from biological age; the latter is noted
by the appearance of specified physiological changes that can truly be
said to appear earlier or later. The chronological meaning of age is, of
course, of little interest to anyone concerned with human, personal
aging.

The desire on the part of biologists to understand the mechanisms and processes that enable a cell line to replicate itself is
certainly worthy of investigation, and we should be clear that, should
they discover the mechanisms which foster such replications, that
outcome could conceivably add to the longevity of the species and its
members. This goal of biological research has led to complaints that
biologists are foolishly conducting "fountain of youth" research. If
this phrase is meant as a disvaluation of such research, it surely
misses the point. For biologists are not searching to uncover the
structure of cellular and subcellular processes in order to keep *young
persons* from becoming *old persons*. That is, they are not trying to
affect personal biography. However, they are intent upon keeping a
typical 80-year-old person *looking like* a 50-year-old person tends to

look. The intent is to discover the mechanisms which govern and limit cell line replication, which is currently thought to be due to intrinsic, "genetically coded" information. For even when cell environments are maintained in optimal nutrient solutions, the number of replications seems to have an intrinsic limit, and the cell line fails to reproduce after a certain, and somewhat constant, number of replications.

Extension of this cellular capacity to reproduce and multiply—keeping in mind our Darwinian heritage—would surely have bearing on the longevity of the species and its members, but it has virtually nothing to do with human personal aging. That is to say, human aging is essentially an historical, experiential, and biographical process, which only persons who experience events and history undergo. In this everyday meaning of aging, cells and genes do not age, though they surely undergo many changes as a function of chronometric time. However, chronometric time alone does not define or describe growing old or being old. The notion of "aging" is not identical to the notion of "change through chronometric time," any more than cellular changes in the facial skin are identical to the meaning of the wrinkled brow of the aged person.

Where biologists should be employing terms like "change" and "chronometry," they often carelessly employ the terms "age" and "aging." A good rule would be the following: if one is referring to changes occurring in measured time (chronometry), one should avoid the terms "age" and "aging" altogether. After all, for many years biologists were quite pleased to argue for the truth of their reductionistic models. Is it not, therefore, now inconsistent for them to reverse their position and apply to the NIA for support for "aging research" since aging, in short, does not occur in cells or organ systems and certainly not within the chromosome? Nevertheless, I suspect that neuroscientists will continue to seek support to study "brain aging" and will continue to report their results as "age-related changes in the brain." But brains do not grow old either. Only people do, people who, of course, "have" brains. We might well say that our dog grows old. But does it really age? To make that a workable expression, we have adopted the myth that the dog's lifetime can be accurately compared to ours such that for every seven of our human years (chronometrically speaking) the dog has one! The absurdity of this suggestion should be obvious. We certainly can't mean that one year of the calendar is equal to seven years of the calendar. Furthermore, we certainly cannot take seriously the suggestion that physiological changes from the human infant's birth date to age seven is an accurate description of what physiologically occurs in the dog by age one. By now it should be clear that a good deal of confusion is generated by the careless application to the biological level of everyday language, which should only have been employed at the personal level of human social life.

It should not require much additional argument to demonstrate that research into the mechanisms of various diseases (e.g., osteoporosis, a thinning of the bone which occurs with late onset, especially in women) is precisely disease research. If certain diseases tend to occur later in the life cycle, their prevention or postponement is not intrinsically a study of aging. Once again, *persons* grow old and age, and it is with this clearly in mind that we intuitively reject the suggestion that young persons with progeria are really old persons, though their external (and some internal) "markers" give them the *appearance* of aged people. But it is an appearance of being old, not a truly old person, that we see. This is clear to us because we ordinarily and properly restrict our notions of "being old" and "aging" to historical and biographical beings.

Another intuitive point is worthy of mention here: In many scientific papers and in the *Special Report on Aging* it is not uncommon to find the terms "age" and "aging" set off by quotation marks. These "scarecrow" marks are frequently employed syntactically to indicate a tongue-in-cheek reference, or to suggest that the reader not take the meaning literally. Hence the *Report* which I mentioned states: "Knowledge of what takes place in cells as they age is vital to an understanding of 'cellular aging' and the aging process in general." The use of quotation marks for the expression "cellular aging" indicates, on behalf of the authors of the *Report,* some discomfort with the notion of cellular aging—that is, 'aging' seems to them inappropriate as a correct description of the biologists' study of cellular changes.

Additional confusion is created by the use of expressions which suggest that aging is both the cause of changes in the body of the person and the result of various physiological processes: "As I age my skin becomes wrinkled" is an expression in which "age" is employed to mean *time passing* and age (time) is taken as the cause of my body's wrinkling. But quite in conflict with the notion of aging as cause of wrinkling and disease is the notion that, as a result of various physiological processes, one becomes old and aged. How is it that aging is both the *cause* of bodily "markers" and disease as well as the *result* of complex changes at the cellular and subcellular levels? How often have physicians offered their patients an "explanation" of their complaints and illnesses which included the sentence: "You have this condition *because* you are old?"

I have already mentioned research on longevity and extended survival and I have argued that such research does not qualify as research in the biology of aging, since the phenomenon of aging is historical. I draw the same conclusion with respect to research on those diseases which are associated with or accompany aged persons. But such diseases, for example, osteoporosis or atherosclerosis are not "inevitable concomitants" of aging. This is a most important point. The study of disease processes, at the cellular and genetic levels, which occur with greater frequency in aged persons—those within the chronological range of 60 to 90 years—is certainly important research, but we should be clear that at this point there obtains, it appears, only a contingent association between senescence and disease onset. Certainly diseases like osteoporosis may one day be prevented or have a postponed onset beyond the maximum or mean life span of the members of the human species (and eventually be eliminated from the species),[17] but that will be the result of biological research into the nature of disease mechanisms, not into aging.

There is a problem here, of course; if the rate of progression of a given disease is decreased, "then the date of passage through the clinical threshold is postponed; if sufficiently postponed," writes James Fries, "the symptomatic threshold may not be closed during a lifetime, and the disease is 'prevented.' "[18] The notion of "prevention" employed here is one of postponement. That is, by the time a disease "D" could get you, you're already dead. Not only is there reason to take joy from this, you may already have lived to a mean age of 85 years. Furthermore, Dr. Fries holds out the false promise of a natural death. You die of old age, and age in the purely objective chronological sense will once again be offered as an explanation of the cause of your "passing." Even more importantly and more correctly, a biological understanding of those disease processes that "accompany" our old age should be called precisely the pathophysiology of "disease processes" and *not* "aging processes." If the latter notion is employed here, it is an easy inference, though surely an incorrect one, to the conclusion that "aging is a disease." One could say, with Sally Gadow, that "the notion that aging is a disease is a disease."

One need only consider the incoherent suggestion offered by Robert R. Kohn in his *Principles of Mammalian Aging,* especially in the chapter entitled "Characteristics of Aging Processes": "Other steadily progressing processes, which are not usually considered to represent aging, are certain diseases. These are referred to as 'diseases' because they occur in only a fraction of a population. If they occurred in all members of a population, they would be called 'aging processes.' " From this Kohn concludes that an aging process is one that "occurs in all members of a population, that is progressive and irreversible under usual conditions, and that begins or accelerates at maturity in those systems which undergo growth and development."[19] In his final chapter he concludes that "it may be difficult to identify a process under observation as an aging one, and to distinguish it from a disease in a certain subgroup."[20]

But at the present time we do not know enough about the relationship between mechanisms of certain diseases (e.g., osteoporosis) to claim that they are more than contingently related (as opposed to necessarily related or causally related) to growing old. If we lack information, if we do not yet understand what is meant by aging processes, then we are unable to make a case for the nature of the relationship between certain diseases and aging. The mistake lies in labeling the process (and the research it generates) as "cellular aging," for we must work to see if/how cellular change in the human organism over time correlates with the perceived manifestations of that human experience we call aging, and then to see if/how these correlate with other processes and mechanisms that have been identified as particular to certain diseases which seem to appear with more regularity in the experience of aged persons.

Much of the current confusion could be eliminated once we understand that 1) aging is not a disease; 2) disease processes which appear in all members of a population need not be called "aging processes"; 3) aging need not be construed as necessarily entailing an irreversibility or degenerative processes; 4) failure to identify a process as a disease does not automatically justify calling the process an "aging process." The distinction needed here is already available: normal vs. pathological processes. Even Kohn remarks that an aging process is "a normal process, in that it occurs in all members of the population under consideration."[21]

To recapitulate: chronological age is measured, quantified time and biologists appropriately apply chronometric measures in their cellular investigations. But aging processes necessarily entail qualitative alterations of personal, historical, and social life.

Finally, it is necessary to offer an account of what biologists study when they inquire into the "markers" or "signs" of aging. Is this properly the arena of the biology of aging? Again, as with longevity and disease research, I suggest that biologists are not inquiring into aging processes. But is not inquiry into the "outer markers"—slowing gait, graying, wrinkling, "age spots" of the sagging and drying skin—truly the biology of aging? Is not the investigation of the "inner markers"—central nervous system changes, decreased muscle strength, and changes in the immune system—the heart of the biology of aging? I think not. The study of the processes undergone by the cells of the aged person's skin, for example, is not an inquiry into wrinkling, but rather a study of epidermal changes over chronos-time. The lines of the face, that is, the full physiognomy of the face of the elderly person is not the *sum* of all facial wrinkles. Why is it we plainly say of the old sea captain that his face reveals, in part, his history and life style? Or recall the richly lined face of an important man of the church, the Canon George van der Peale, a detail of the larger painting "Madonna of the Canon van der Peale" painted by the Flemish artist Jon van Eyck in 1436.[22]

In short, do we really add to our understanding of human aging when we allow ourselves to accept the claim of biologists that their dermatological studies are studies in "dermatological senescence"? Each aged human face is a contextual totality in which is expressed a specific and unique personal history. Biologists should remain silent at this level of meaning. One day, of course, the physiological sciences may discover how to prevent the onset of diseases and the "markers" or "signs" of aging, but that event will in no way lead to the conclusion that young people will be kept from becoming old people. What will be true at this future time is the claim that *old people will appear as young people now do;* and when this day comes we will have no "outer markers" of aging with which to judge a person's chronological age and, more importantly, no way to judge easily the unique and long personal history which that old person embodies. We can, if we wish, encourage the biological scientist to discover how to conceal or prevent aging of the skin; after all, as Murphy and Gastel of the NIA remind us, "changes in the skin are among the most common, apparent, and *distressing* signs of aging" and our culture assigns a positive value only to a "youthful integument."[23] Where, if at all, then, can we discover the positive valuations of aging and the aged when it is clear that biology will never in principle offer such an account?

Conclusion: Transcending the Biological Approach to Aging

In his essay "The Historical Developments in the Biological Aspects of Aging and the Aged," Alfred H. Lawton paraphrased L. du Nuoy (viz. *Human Destiny*): "The more deeply the biologist analyzed, the further he seemed to remove himself from the problem he meant to solve. The details he studied prevent the recapture of a concept of the unified problem."[24] My thesis is more radical than Dr. Lawton's, however. Whereas he remains content with the notion of "biological research in aging," I have tried to argue that we should deny the conceptual legitimacy of this formulation of what biologists in fact investigate.

Lawton, however, is at least correct in his criticism that "as gerontology matured as a true subspecialty of biology, there developed those geniuses, the superspecialists. The very nature of their preoccupation with engrossing detail tends to cause them to lose sight of the total problem of understanding aging."[25] My thesis denies that biological research can ever be research in aging, and hence it follows that biologists need not agonize about aging any more or less than the rest of us. That is, as aging persons we should attend to the time of the *curriculum vitae,* to the temporality of our very personal senescence. Each person's life history is that for which he can be praised or blamed; it is constituted by events, decisions, and turning points, accomplishments, failures, acute and chronic illnesses, and so on. It is what *should* emerge after "taking" a history of, say, the geriatric patient.

The standpoint I have suggested, then, has as its foundation the fact that the contemporary biological perspective on aging is a logical extension of Darwinism. It is promulgated in the axiomatic truths of biology—for example, that the life span of our species (as well as others) is genetically determined and that (as the biologist would have it) the processes of aging in our species as well as others is due to an "accumulation of genetic error,"[26] generated by somatic mutations (mutations in accord with the laws that govern randomness).

Such "axiomatic truths" of biology, however, intrinsically entail a conceptual and negatively-evaluative model of aging persons. Namely, true aging is viewed as the result of degeneration and decline in functional capacity. With decline comes decreased integument, increased vulnerability and a slow accumulation of deteriorative, multiform irreparable changes equated with eventual *loss.* This is the negative-evaluative paradigm, even if some biologists, like Zhores S. Medvedev (who conducts what should be called research on longevity), are careful to point out that "aging is multiform at all levels of biological organization" and that all attempts by biologists to discover a single process of aging or to "create the universal theory of aging" are "simplistic."[27]

The biological language of aging is negatively value-laden (instead of purely descriptive) and the application of this language to the history, experience, and perception of the human person is unwarranted. It is a valuation that is not only metaphysically in-appropriate but morally inappropriate, in that it implies certain things with respect to personhood (and respect for persons) that are quite negative. These moral implications may well be very far-reaching and for that reason ought to be grounded in a less arbitrary, less controversial, and nonnegative, value-laden description.

It is one of the aims of the humanities, taken collectively, to uncover the value of the full range of human experience. The biolo-gical perspective on aging reveals, at best, only half-truths. For the essence of senescence is not captured by notions like "failure to transmit progeny," "failure to repair subcellular DNA structures," or "failure to replicate germ cell lines." Such pervasive, negative valua-tions not only reflect a "humanistic disequilibrium," but easily serve to bias the young clinician in whose care the aging and elderly will find themselves. The aging person is a complex being-in-the-world. To more fully understand aging persons, then, we do not really need further biological explanations, but rather a complete phenomenolo-gical description of the experience of growing old.

Regrettably, not only has the biological paradigm of devaluation dominated the scene for the last century, but even the most eminent biologists, like Sir MacFarlane Burnet, have fallen into the trap. In his *Intrinsic Mutagenesis: A Genetic Approach to Aging,* Burnet remarks that, "The most important correlate of aging is death."[28] No longer is the most important correlate of aging "the loss of capacity to reproduce"; now aging is "just a poor second choice to dying young."[29] It is a very short step from such remarks about aging to constant talk of death, as if death and dying were only appropriated by the senes-cent members of the community.

But aging, in truth, is not a disease, nor is it a syndrome, or *"maladie obscure,"* to borrow a phrase from the poet, Eustache Deschamps.[30] The impact of such thinking for those who are re-sponsible for health care for the aging and aged is, in my view, profound indeed. In conclusion, dialogue between geriatricians, phi-losophers, and other humanists has not occurred with sufficient fre-quency or regularity. Our era has not witnessed a serious, formal engagement between philosophers and those professionals who care for the infirm elderly. I am hopeful, however, that with the rise of geriatric medicine and a slow increase in the number of geriatric physicians who attend to the very aged, this dialogue may well take place more frequently in the future. There is, of course, the ever-present danger that geriatricians and philosophers will talk past one another. That would indeed be unfortunate; for we should be re-minded that physicians and other health professionals who care for the infirm aged have not received a philosophical education, and only a very few philosophers have been formally trained in medicine, however refined their sentiments and impeccable their sense of justice and equity.

Furthermore, the education of physicians is, since Abraham Flexner's famous report, essentially scientific, that is, a biological and physiological enterprise, with special attention being paid to subcellular phenomena. In our scientific-technological era the ancient riddle—"Thou hast been considering whether the chicken came first from the egg or the egg from the chicken?"—first raised by Macrobius, circa 400 A.D.,[31] has, of course, been resolved (the egg came first), not only by Darwin's theory of heritability and later accounts of mutation, but by the seminal work of Watson and Crick prior to 1953,[32] anticipated by Samuel Butler in 1877: Recall the latter's famous aphorism: "A hen is only an egg's way of making another egg." The latest reformulation might be: "A human being is only DNA's way of making more DNA."

The profound dehumanization of such microcosmic images of mankind and aged persons suggests, to say the least, that we have now placed the accent on the very edges of life—I mean eggs, genes, and DNA—and have thereby come very close indeed to describing, if not defining, ourselves, especially our aging selves, out of existence.

Postscript

Having taken the time to argue for the thesis that biologists do not study aging, a few interesting consequences can be derived from this thesis: First, the National Institute on Aging, in funding the research of biologists, may have sustained—without intent of course—a national hoax. Biologists who are, especially today, more and more desperate for federal support to pursue their hypotheses, have been pleased to apply for and receive the largesse made possible by our tax dollars directed to research on aging, I mean the "biology of aging" (a phrase I now place in quotation marks to indicate a clearly pejorative tone). Scientists of integrity do not hesitate to admit (at least when queried privately) that the "biology of aging" grant line has simply made possible research they would have previously placed, and correctly so, under "disease research," or "longevity" research, and so forth. Since these scientists are typically committed to what Hans Jonas calls the "internal norms of scientific inquiry"—they are careful in their work, keep faith with the standards of science, acknowledge the value of truth, are usually dedicated, persistent, disciplined, open-minded and tend to share their results with the scientific community—I have no quarrel with them, though the federal research rubrics are highly suspicious, since every dollar directed to the "biology of aging" is a dollar *not* directed to the care of the infirm elderly.

But what does it mean to emphasize, at the national level, care of the infirm elderly? Certainly such care requires the continued availability of competent medical personnel. And where is that competence obtained? Obviously, through the long and arduous educational and training programs conducted by American medical and health professional schools. And how, given the multiple pressures to forestall the establishment of a subspecialty in geriatric medicine in this country, are we to assure ourselves that students of medicine, nursing, and the other health professions will be confronted with an appropriate curriculum and training program in geriatric medicine and geriatric care? The answer is, regrettably, already predetermined: Medical students, for example, spend two years studying biology—including normal and pathological processes. And since these two scientifically-oriented years are always propaedeutic to the advanced two clinical years, the obvious answer is that if we are going to produce competent health professionals to care for the elderly in the clinical context, then we shall have to introduce these same students to geriatric principles in the first two years of medical school. And that, of course, means they must be introduced to the biology of aging.

The second consequence of my argument, then, is that we must form a conspiracy: we should tell no one of my argument, especially if it is sound. For the practical and dangerous consequence of my view is that medical students may *never* achieve clinical competence in the care of the elderly, the absence of which is already a national crisis, and which surely will be exacerbated by the end of this century if things remain as they are at present. This "conspiracy" is required, since the care of the elderly in the United States is far more important than the arguments of this philosopher or perhaps any philosopher. So care of the indigent, infirm aged among us remains a duty beyond the duty to disseminate the truth, however nontrivial that truth might be. Am I advocating hypocrisy? I think not. As much as I would like to be right (and have others agree with me), the price is too dear for those for whom life itself is extremely precious. I am left with more questions in this regard, and wonder whether this, what I recommend, is a form of what Hans Jonas has called the "practical uses of theory." Frankly I doubt it. Rather, it is the giving way of theory to ethical praxis, a radical alteration of values with which contemporary philosophers too may have to cope. When our tax dollars are directed to research in the "biology of aging," let's keep the faith. For only by remaining silent about this national hoax can we reasonably assure ourselves that the infirm elderly among us have a hope of access to competent health care while they live out their penultimate years, months, and days.

Notes

[1]James F. Fries, "Aging, Natural Death, and the Compression of Morbidity," *The New England Journal of Medicine* 303 (July 17, 1980): 130–135.

[2]*Senescence: The Last Half of Life* (New York: D. Appleton and Co., 1922), p. vii.

[3]This point, which I owe to Professor Edward J. Kollar, is of central importance in understanding the negative influence of Darwinism on current attitudes toward the elderly. Also see Gene Bylinsky's "Science is on the Trail of the Fountain of Youth," *Fortune* 94, (July 1976), reprinted in the *Congressional Record—House* (July 29, 1976), p. 8009. Bylinsky observes that, "to put it bluntly, nature has little interest in the survival of the individual members of a species once they have had time to give birth to and rear their young." (p. 8009)

[4]François Jacob, *The Logic of Life* (New York: Pantheon Books, Random House, 1973), pp. 17, 20.

[5]Bernard L. Strehler, *Time, Cells, and Aging* (2nd ed.) (New York: Academic Press, 1977), p. 11.

[6]———. pp. 11–12.

[7]Donald G. Murphy, and Barbara Gastel, "National Institute on Aging and Dermatologic Research," *Journal of the American Academy of Dermatology* 2 (April, 1980): 341.

[8]Joseph T. Freeman, "Kiev to Kiev in Gerontology: 1938–1972," *The Gerontologist* 13 (Winter 1973): 404.

[9]Strehler, *Time, Cells, and Aging*, p. 16.

[10]Michael Rose, and Brian Charlesworth, "A Test of Evolutionary Theories of Senescence," *Nature* 287 (September 11, 1980): 141.

[11]———.

[12]Strehler, *Time, Cells, and Aging*, p. 31.

[13]———. p. 35.

[14]*Special Report on Aging, 1980* (Bethesda, Maryland: U.S. Department of Health and Human Services) (PHS, NIH, NIA) NIH Publication No. 80–2135, August 1980, p. 21.

[15]———. My emphasis.

[16]*Ibid.*

[17]Fries, *Compression of Morbidity*, pp. 130–135.

[18]_____. p. 133.

[19]Robert R. Kohn, *Principles of Mammalian Aging* (Englewood Cliffs, NJ: Prentice-Hall, 1971), p. 9. Also see Kohn's "Biomedical Aspects of Aging," in *Aging, Death, and the Completion of Being*, David D. Van Tassel, ed. (Philadelphia: University of Pennsylvania Press, 1979), pp. 3, 5.

[20]Kohn, p. 164.

[21]Kohn, p. 9.

[22]Geri Berg, and Sally Gadow, "Toward More Human Meanings of Aging: Ideals and Images From Philosophy and Art," in *Aging and the Elderly: Humanistic Perspective in Gerontology*, Stuart F. Spicker, K. M. Woodward and D. D. Van Tassel, eds. (Atlantic Highlands, NJ: Humanities Press, 1978), pp. 87–88 and Plate 2. Also see Freeman's "Kiev to Kiev" in *Gerontology, op. cit.*, p. 406. Here one finds a typical discussion of the anatomy of skin research. Note that the only language used is relatively negatively value-laden. Terms like "degeneration," "dissolution," "atrophy," and "cell diminution" are always employed. Such value-laden accounts are the only ones available at the level of physiology and anatomy.

[23]D. G. Murphy, and B. Gastel, "Dermatologic Research," p. 341. My emphasis.

[24]*The Gerontologist* 5, 1, Part II, (March, 1965): 31. My italics.

[25]_____.

[26]Sir MacFarlane Burnet, *Intrinsic Mutagenesis: A Genetic Approach to Aging*, (New York-Toronto: John Wiley & Sons 1974), p. vii.

[27]"Aging and Longevity," *The Gerontologist* 15 (June 1975): 198. Also see Medvedev's "Error Theories of Aging," *Alternstheorien: Zellkernmembranen*, D. Platt, (ed.) (Stuttgart-New York: F. K. Schattauer Verlag, 1976), pp. 37–46.

[28]Sir MacFarlane Burnet, *Intrinsic Mutagenesis*, p. 50.

[29]Robert Kastenbaum, "Exit and Existence: Society's Script for Old Age and Death," in *Aging, Death, and the Completion of Being*. This remark appeared in the original manuscript, read during the "Human Values and Aging" project at Case Western Reserve University (November 1975), p. 27.

[30]Simone de Beauvior, *The Coming of Age*, Patrick O'Brien, trans., (New York, Warner Paperbacks, 1973), p. 218.

[31]*Saturnalia*, VII, xvi.

[32]"Molecular Structure of Nucleic Acids," *Nature* 171 (April 25, 1953): 737–738.

4

Transitions and Imperatives
In Long-term Care

MICHAEL J. STOTTS

Introduction

Long-term care for older adults represents a major health delivery subsystem in this country, but it is an area of our human services system which is underdeveloped, understudied, underresearched, and little understood by families and patients who are directly involved with it. Because an increasing number of people are touched by long-term care,[1] there would seem to be an emphasis on rationalizing policies, regulations, and sanctions which have as their basis the design of a continuum of services which improves on presently fragmented support systems. While a multitude of responsibilities have been undertaken by the federal government (with limited support from the private sector) there is as yet no consensus about the development of policy for long-term care. The following discussion suggests some benchmarks for planning and may help to illustrate what lies ahead in this decade.

The development of policies and actions by the principal decision makers in long-term care must not continue to isolate services normally identified as mainstream programs, such as hospitals, mental health centers, university medical centers, and health maintenance clinics. Further divisions occur if we continue to label programs for older people as institutional vs. noninstitutional.

Because most of the attention has been on the nursing home as the leading provider of institutional care for older people, we have neglected the development of other support systems. By broadening the perspective to include a variety of services, not all of which are health services, our future decisions in long-term care should not reinforce unevenness but, instead, should include a more global approach with emphasis on the client, delivery of the service, and on the quality of the actual care received.

Consider briefly the following dispositions which are characteristic of policy and practices in the recent past: (1) The implementation of policy has reflected a strong preoccupation with the nursing home as representing "an ideal" way to care for older people. Demonstration of this policy is best illustrated in Medicare and Medicaid legislation; (2) We recognize that the nursing home as the principal institutional provider of skilled and intermediate care for older adults demands our attention and our resources, mainly to correct inequities and inadequacies which have been largely neglected in the past; Our efforts to bring stability and higher quality of care into nursing homes should not consume our limited energies and resources; (3) Our health and human services agencies have initially ignored and consequently left to chance the development of other service systems. It might even be observed that policy initiatives have been heavily biased toward institutional care, placing emerging alternate systems at a severe disadvantage. Further, there is little evidence that linkages, integrative mechanisms, or "long-term care systems" are desirable goals.

It is quite possible to leave well enough alone, to continue in the present direction, following a course which may accomplish the greatest good for the greatest number, but our resources are limited, while both costs and demand for services are increasing.[2] To continue on course without substantial changes in policy reformulation will only increase the total bill for health care for older people and may conceivably limit the options which are open to us, at least in the short run. Cosmetic changes in policy, as was the case in the recent Medicare amendments (passed in the "eleventh hour" of the 96th Congress and in the 1982 tax bill appropriations and budget reconciliation bills) only put off larger, more encompassing decisions which are inevitable.

Alternatives

The issue of alternatives to nursing home care has been superseded in health policy parlance by other catch phrases, but the goal is the same: To create and develop services for older people which are not limited to institutional care. As a recent position paper pointed out, the question of institutional vs. noninstitutional care for the elderly has been debated for a long time.[3] It is unlikely that we have seen an end to a continuing concern with this topic until cost, quality, and equity factors are defined more precisely.

Alternatives to hospital and nursing home care first received national attention, both by the public and by health and social services professionals, after President Nixon made a speech at the Greenbriar Nursing Home in Nashua, New Hampshire, in 1971. In that policy statement, the federal government was committed to a course of action which would apply a significant amount of resources to solving the problems of overutilization and substandard care in the nation's nursing homes. The intent of this program, called "The Nursing Home Improvement Program," was, in part, to construct alternatives to institutionalization by testing other ways in which to care for older people.[4]

Innovations

Another approach to the discovery of viable alternatives was to encourage the creation of innovative models of service delivery and the demonstration of new ways by which older people could have adequate access to health and social services. This became the announced policy of the federal government in its search for improved methods for dealing with burgeoning cost problems and consumer dissatisfaction with the limited options open to them. Section 222 of the 1972 Social Security Amendments authorized a number of demonstrations which featured day care services under Title XVIII and XIX and, particularly, Part B of Title XVIII. Essentially, this was a "crash program" by the federal government to provide resources which would identify new information about costs of day care and how this service might be shown to help older people stay out of institutions as long as possible. The Section 222 demonstrations were intended to contain, that is, limit, the systematic institutionalization of people in homes of one kind or another, and to show that there are other viable methods of caring for older people with chronic and disabling conditions. From those many experiments came a renewed emphasis in the development of long-term care programs and systems in home health, day care, and a diverse number of innovative services.[5]

Parallel Services

The concept of parallel services is one described by Hammerman[6] and elaborated into a human service model in a report by the Subcommittee on Human Services of the House Select Committee on Aging.[7] The fundamental principle embodied in parallel services is choice of services which, within reasonable limits, can be selected by purchasers of care. Home health services, for example, have been clearly shown to be an effective health delivery system for chronically ill older people. This shift in policy may be observed to include such parallel services not only as home care but day care, respite care, and hospice care. This is best reflected in health and fiscal policies under Medicare and Medicaid, which are now broadening their coverages and entitlements for the elderly. This broadened financing, consequently, has softened the federal government's bias towards institutionalized care. As parallel services, home-health day care, and variations of these models should be available alongside institutional care. The human service model, described by the House Committee, reviews several possible approaches which are identified as required for elders, that is, those adults 75 years and older;[8] but it is firm in its recommendation for a full "floor of services."

Considerations in Defining the Problem

Because the long-term care institution in our society is highly visible and probably the most entrenched program in long-term care, it has been increasingly difficult to replace or interface the institution with other programs. Hammerman[9] sees the institution as a program that has a great deal to offer, but its visibility, easy access, and the relative lack of other community resources have resulted in a maldistribution of institutional services, a generally expensive program, and a unidimensional approach to providing a system of patient care for older people. Simultaneously, the institution has not been provided the incentives (or permitted by legislative authority) to realize its own potential to deliver services beyond its front door nor to develop a flexibility in its program which would encourage the public to use its expertise in any other way than to participate in its fulltime care program.

Whichever way the problem is approached, a continuum of services seems to be secondary to a Medicare policy that rigidifies the system as follows: the patient goes to the hospital, then to the skilled nursing facility, and finally to home care services. In most cases the care is apportioned on the basis of its intensity and, as Shore points out, on the quality of care often measured in terms of quantity.[10] Shore argues for a more comprehensive public policy by showing that the emphasis has been on the quality of care when it should be, instead, on the quality of life. He maintains that we have a two-tiered approach to constructing programs for older people in this country. The fundamental assumption that drives this policy rests on a belief that "people are either well and primarily in need of income supports or they are generally sick and in need of intensive medical care." A client-centered policy to long-term care would obviate this fragmentation and challenge the assumptions which continue to impede a more unified public policy, that is, the delivery of services that are so often inseparable: medical, social, and mental care.

What considerations should be incorporated into any concerted approaches to the solution of major problems of cost, quality, access, choice, and equity in health care for older people? Can a formulated approach be developed which meets the diverse constituent needs of clients, purchasers of care, and providers of services, and which delivers health services to the community efficiently? The position taken here is that we have done well, considering that the modern long-term care systems that we have are mainly post-Medicare. In this short time, much has been accomplished, but our policy has been mainly caretaking and not very vigorous in effecting changes in the existing patterns of service, for example, toward preventive care.

Some examples of considerations which should be taken into account in construction of policy directions include:

1. The allocation and reallocation of resources, both human and financial, are major undertakings. The expertise to care for older people with chronic health conditions is largely found in long-term care institutions. Not only are the personnel employed in these institutions, but they exist like the institution itself, that is, away from the mainstream of health care. Attempts to reorganize, redirect, or reallocate these important resources are uncommonly difficult problems.

2. There is little evidence to document what full-time, long-term care can do for a person in need of services. Consequently, what part-time care can do is largely unknown. Related to this issue are the roles of the family, volunteers, and friends as participants in part-time care systems that are devised. In addition, there is the

issue of any interface between full-time care systems (long-term care institutions) and part-time care systems, such as home health.

3. Institutional programs already have a privileged and entrenched position. Alternate support systems which are not institutionally-grounded cannot always be justified because they are a "better mousetrap." The process by which one shows consequential differences in alternate schemes of care require the participation of several providers. Most institutional nursing home programs are controlled by proprietary interests. These homes are not inclined to participate in research that may ultimately give a competitor a better edge. Competition for patients is a major objective of proprietary and most nonprofit organizations, and this competition alone creates a barrier to cooperative enterprises.

4. The population to be served is difficult to identify. On the one hand are very dependent, older people who some say can only properly be cared for in institutions. On the other hand, there is a very large proportion of older people who would prefer to remain independent, if they had some supplemental support which would assist them in continuing their present lifestyles. Somewhere in between are the services which are increasingly being commended to the well and frail elderly and which provide services within a larger system that can respond supportively toward the prevention of institutionalization.

5. Certainly the total cost of service must be carefully described in contrast to what has been too frequently a comparison of per diem costs. Per diem cost is only one way to measure the costs of services for older people. Studies must begin to emphasize a more global view of the cost problem, including many variables which have often been omitted in comparative studies of home health and nursing home costs. Hospital costs for older people are not compared with nursing home costs, for example; nor do hospital costs, comparatively speaking, seem to be in question at all. Similarly, it is counterproductive to compare nursing home and home health care costs. If the goals and benefits of any of these services could be clearly defined, then perhaps we could have a better understanding of what kinds of care are being purchased, what outcomes are being considered, and what are truly the weaknesses and strengths of the various systems of care.

6. Services are increasingly being delivered to older people in their homes. The questions which are being asked include: When does the home service become unnecessary? Will eight hours of home care service per week be sufficient to accomplish a medical, social, or psychological objective, or are six hours sufficient? What services

should families provide? Should families be reimbursed in any way for services? How do we know that a certain service is appropriate for one person? When does that service cease to be useful to the person or carry a markedly diminishing return?

7. Can a single organization effectively administer a mix of services, that include medical, social, and mental health services? Will the present informal networks and sometimes competing organizations be allowed to continue what many believe is a fragmented, inefficient long-term care delivery model which frequently is unable to serve the client well?

This partial list of considerations presents a set of challenges for health personnel, researchers, and policy makers. Problems which are named here are often recognized by personnel who are administering programs. However, geography, distance, ability to pay for services by the client, political and cultural history of the community, and availability of community resources present additional factors that are basic to the application of policies in any one location. In fact, policy implementation is most often under the jurisdiction of several state and community agencies. This is as true at the federal level as it is at state level. The result is too frequently a certain paralysis in effecting change. Coordination and development of fiscal policies, that are consonant with programmatic goals within separately administered agencies, exemplify the counterproductive discontinuity.

Summary of Major Policy Junctures

The accompanying chart chronicles the major policy-related events in long-term care of the Johnson-through-Reagan administrations (Figure 4–1). From a historical viewpoint, the federal government has applied considerable resources and effort toward formulating a long-term care system. Admittedly, the directions appear somewhat circuitous and often only in response to a series of crises (nursing home fires, fraud and corruption by profiteers, exposés of poor and abusive treatment of older people enrolled in entitlement programs). The fact remains that in a relatively short time great strides have been made in implementing policy, particularly health policy, for older people. During the 1980s, we can expect to see a continuation of a trend and to refine the major efforts that have their origins in the policy-related events of the late 1960s and 1970s.

Figure 4–1. Chronology of major federal policy events in long-term care (1965–1982)

1965	Passage of the Social Security Amendments (Medicare/Medicaid) • The Older American's Act
1967	Senate Sub-Committee on Long-term Care established; public hearings begun Social Security Amendments (Kennedy and Moss amendments)—first of contemporary reforms to focus on institutional care standards
1969–1975	Hearings (including a prolific publication of hearings, reports, and recommendations) by the Senate Sub-committee on Long-term Care (oversight activities 1976 to present)
1970	National Advisory Council on Nursing Home Administration presents final recommendations: Codification of long-term care practice published in Federal Register and incorporated into administrator licensure laws
1971	Second White House Conference on Aging; significant recommendations in areas related to health, nursing homes, and access to services by older people
1971–1975	Tenure of the Long-term Care for the Elderly Research Review and Advisory Committee, a multifunctional committee which advised and recommended funding for DHEW initiatives
1972	President Nixon's major policy speech at Nashua, New Hampshire; officially launches the nursing home improvement program • Social Security Amendments of 1972 included extensive changes in Medicare and Medicaid services; significant additional requirements for long-term care institutions • Office of Nursing Home Affairs created in the Office of the Secretary of DHEW (1972–1976)
1974	First of the Senate's widely-distributed 12-volume report summarizing the weaknesses of the long-term care system and the major providers of care • House of Representatives Select Committee on Aging created • Department of Health, Education, and Welfare began a national four-part long-term care improvement campaign focused on the nursing home
1976–1980	Carter Administration dissolves Public Health Service long-term care program efforts; centralizes several activities in a new Health Care Financing Administration • Administration on Aging assumes a lead position in long-term care
1981	Third White House Conference on Aging; Mini-Conferences and similar state activities (1980–1981) focus on federal and state policy formulation
1982	Reagan Administration consolidates long-term care programs begun under Carter; 30,000 board and care homes selected for improved safety and supervision

It may be presumptive to summarize present policy directions, but clearly there is a growing recognition by offices in the bureaucracy and legislators at state and federal levels that the problems of older people who are dependent upon our health and social service programs are politically real, that costs are a constant source of concern, and that experience tells us that governmental supervision, intervention, and leadership are indispensable. How do these and other factors that impinge on policy become translated into action programs? Perhaps a review of some major developmental policy directions will provide insight into what to expect from this decade's legislation and government-sponsored initiatives.

One major initiative is a predisposition to centralize at the local level what could be described as "near total control of the patient." A number of compelling arguments and some demonstrations of "triage" show that if older people are to be well-served by locally-based but separately incorporated agencies, some one person (perhaps, in Britain for example, the British medical officer of health) or one agency (the Regional or State Office on Aging) should be accountable. Research and demonstration in long-term care has been consciously orchestrated by the federal government toward resolving the acknowledged gaps which are judged to be important in effecting such a policy. Consequently, the Health Care Financing Administration and the Administration on Aging are currently funding what has become known as "*the* channeling agency demonstration program." The participation in a leadership capacity of a state agency is a prerequisite of this program. The objective is to test methods of data collection and to coordinate service schemes. Twelve states have received awards.[11]

Secondly, there is also a growing recognition that strict adherence to a medical service delivery model (particularly under the sponsorship of an organization) without long-term care expertise does not adequately meet the requirements or needs of older people *even if they are sick*. This has been a major cause of failure in program development in the long-term care network. The progressive nursing home is an example of one provider that has integrated parallel elements of health care and psychosocial components. This melding of complex care components is very much underdeveloped and most difficult to put into effect. The concepts of interdisciplinary approaches, team care, and the therapeutic community do exist in service programs, but infrequently.

A third imperative appears to be the creation of legislation and policy action groups at the federal and state levels that emphasize new units of organization and that more nearly ensure cooperation between social and health programs for older adults. The synchronization of programs, activities, and policy statements on topics of long-term care has been a constant source of irritation in the federal government. At the state level there is also great division in the supervision of programs which affect older people, that is, health, welfare, and social services. Increasingly, there are examples of state and federal governments merging into one program the various services that affect the aged. For example, Kansas has centralized authority in a cabinet-level Department of Aging; several state governments have had study commissions, executive initiatives aimed at reforming the delivery system, and various advisory and task-identification groups. In the Office of the Secretary in the Department of Health and Human Services, there has been continuous attention to long-term care policy options through the Office of Nursing Home Affairs established in 1971, which was discontinued in the Carter administration. More recently a task force on long-term care headed by an assistant secretary for planning and evaluation acted as a policy-making body without benefit of a long-term care or nursing home "czar."[12]

Another, more wide-ranging, but uncoordinated policy initiative has been and continues to be education and training for long-term health care.[13] Historically, the Public Health Service has assumed this responsibility, and at the present time there are at least two major projects in the Health Resources Administration designed to increase the clinical skills of medical and nursing students who will eventually care for older adults. A less vigorous program includes the geriatric fellowships which are awarded to medical schools by the National Institute on Aging as faculty development incentives. The Administration on Aging in the past has funded a few programs that are intended to provide gerontologic education opportunities for medical and health students. As yet, however, no coordinated strategy to reach the several thousands of health and medical students now in various stages of preparation for practice has been inaugurated; nor are the present efforts more than experimental. A summary of activity in federal manpower policy is contained in a report compiled by the Administration on Aging.[14] This compendium of information demonstrates what issues remain unresolved and offers some suggestions for responding to specific needs.

Previous attempts to mobilize national associations toward upgrading the care given to older adults through manpower training and retraining were sponsored by the Public Health Service from

1970 to 1976. These efforts had a salutory effect in professional retraining programs. Except for nursing, which now has several programs with an emphasis in gerontology, there has been less than an enthusiastic response by baccalaureate and graduate programs in allied health and medical schools to self-initiate special curriculum design efforts. Manpower retraining and inservice programs in the field of long-term care generally cannot be underestimated as a necessary adjunct to other educational efforts in the professions.

Finally, there is the growing public recognition that the long-term care system we do have is less than perfect. To change direction (away from the Medicare/Medicaid model, for example) is almost to create a new fabric out of whole cloth. In one lengthy review of alternatives, Kahana and Coe admit to no ready answers.[15] Much of the research, they point out, has been designed with various policy-related considerations in mind: spiraling costs, age segregation concerns, roles of families, administration of services, and consumer participation in the process of decision-making. Little attention has been given to the needs of the client or research posited from the perspective of the client. In a new "floor of services" recommended by the House Committee on Aging, what are the expectations about those services? What is their breadth and depth? What is the appropriateness of these services, and how will decisions be made about them? Unidimensional and unidisciplinary research will not satisfactorily resolve a multidimensional problem when applied to an interdisciplinary area such as long-term care.

As noted above, a number of demonstration and innovative programs have been devised. In the Pennsylvania Domiciliary Care Program and New York's Nursing Home Without Walls, alternative institutional roles in care are being tested. Triage in Connecticut and the Community Care Organization (CCO) in Wisconsin are predicated on the basis that efficiency can be replicated[16] by unifying administration of diverse services under the direction of one community-based organization. Such wide-ranging experiments, in part, are designed to demonstrate a state responsibility in a continuum of long-term care services.

Conclusion

There should be no argument about the transitional state of long-term care or the system of health and social services designed for older adults. How this system is perceived by a variety of public policy makers is another question. In health, we often speak of a professional perspective as in a medical or a nursing model. In long-term care, generally, the model has not yet been created. Where a concept of long-term care has been developed locally, the model has not been effectively communicated to a larger audience. The goals of care, that is, rehabilitative, maintenance, protective, or support, have likewise not been universally agreed upon. For minority populations, the rural poor, and the older adult in sixth-floor city walk-ups, the problems are magnified two- or three-fold. Consequently, the expected outcomes are virtually unknown. Studies on the efficacy of management of the patient in controlled situations with chronically ill, older people are almost nonexistent. All of the ambiguity which surrounds our system of care for older adults in need must be dealt with more systematically, with greater vigor, and with more dedication than has historically been evident in federal and state governments.

Notes

[1] Herman Brotman, *Every Ninth American,* Senate Special Committee on Aging, Washington, D.C. U.S. Government Printing Office (1980).

[2] American Health Care Association, *Long-Term Facts,* Washington, D.C., American Health Care Association (1975) and U.S. Department of Health, Education, and Welfare, *Health United States 1979,* Washington, D.C. U.S. Government Printing Office (1980).

[3] Carl C. Pegels, "Institutional vs. Noninstitutional Care for the Elderly," *Journal of Health Policy, Politics and Law* 5 (Summer 1980): pp. 205–212.

[4] U.S. Department of Health, Education, and Welfare, *Long-Term Care Facility Improvement Study,* Washington, D.C. U.S. Government Printing Office, (1975), pp. 1–2 and 69–74.

[5] Day care has grown from 15 programs in 1974 to over 600 in 1980. Home health agencies under voluntary or public auspices have remained about the same (approximately 2,500), but proprietary home care agencies have increased dramatically. Hospice care has also developed rapidly and coordinated service brokers, such as Triage, Inc., in Plainville, Connecticut, have demonstrated the value of a single entry system for adult health and support services. For a discussion of home health and day care programs, see: U.S. Congress, House Select Committee on Aging, *Adult Day Care Programs, Hearings Before a Subcommittee on Health and Long-Term Care,* 96th Congress, 2d sess. (1980) and U.S. Congress, Senate, Special Committee on Aging, *Hearings on Health*

Care for Older Americans: The "Alternatives" Issue, Part 2, 95th Congress, 1st sess. (1977).

[6]Jerome Hammerman, "The Role of the Institution and the Concept of Parallel Services," *The Gerontologist* 14 (February 1974): pp. 11–12. See also Hammerman's "Health Services: Their Success and Failure in Reaching Older Adults," *American Journal of Public Health* 64 (March 1974): 253–256.

[7]U.S. Congress, House Select Committee on Aging, *Future Directions for Aging Policy: A Human Service Model,* 96th Cong. 2d sess., 1980, pp. 2–8.

[8]————. p.4.

[9]Hammerman, "The Role of the Institution," p. 12.

[10]Herbert Shore, "Public Policy for Long Term Care," *Long Term Care and Health Services Administration Quarterly* (Fall, 1980), pp. 242–243.

[11]The states awarded channeling grants are: Florida, Kentucky, Maine, Maryland, Massachusetts, Wisconsin, New Jersey, New York, Ohio, Pennsylvania, and Texas.

[12]Patricia R. Harris, *Memorandum on Task Force on Long Term Care,* U.S. Department of Health, Education, and Welfare, Washington, D.C., Office of the Secretary (December 3, 1979).

[13]Education and training needs have been cited in several reports. One of the most comprehensive is a recent report of a study which focuses on medical school curriculum but has implications for the entire field of long-term care. Robert Kane et al., *Geriatrics in the United States: Manpower Projections and Training Considerations* (Santa Monica, CA: The Rand Corporation, 1980), pp. 63–70.

[14]U.S. Department of Health and Human Services, *A Preliminary Report on the Development and Implementation of a Federal Manpower Policy for the Field of Aging,* Washington, D.C., Office of Human Development Services, Administration on Aging (September 30, 1980).

[15]E. Kahana, and R. M. Coe, "Alternatives in Long-Term Care," in S. Sherwood (ed.), *Long-Term Care: A Handbook for Researchers, Planners, and Providers* (New York: Spectrum Publications, Inc., 1975).

[16]Many of the experimental designs appear as descriptions of innovative programs in hearings of the Senate and House Committees quoted above. Other references are: Gerald M. Eggert, Joyce E. Bowlyow, and Carol W. Nichols, "Gaining Control of the Long-Term Care System: First Returns from the ACCESS Experiment," *The Gerontologist* 20 March 1980, 356–363; U.S. Department of Health, Education, and Welfare, "Nursing Homes Without Walls in New York State," in *Perspectives* by Constance Rhoades-Warden and Jack Knowlton, Washington, D.C., Health Care Financing Administration, November 1980, pp. 5–22; *Triage: Coordinated Services to the Elderly* (Plainville, Connecticut, Triage), n.d.; Joan Quinn, Joan Segal, Helen Raisz, and Christine Johnson, *Coordinating Community Services for the Elderly* (New York: Springer Publishing Co., 1982).

5

Medical Care of the Institutionalized Aged: A Scottish-American Comparison

JEANIE S. KAYSER-JONES

Since the beginning of the twentieth century, the number and proportion of the elderly in the United Kingdom and in the United States have continued to rise steadily; both countries, in common with other industrialized societies, face similar issues in attempting to solve the medical and social problems of old age. Although the problems are similar, Britain and the United States have taken rather different paths in their approach to the care of the aged. In the late 1940s geriatrics was established as a specialty in Britain, and both acute- and long-term care of the aged has become an integral part of the health care structure, whereas, in the United States, geriatrics is not a specialty, and chronic, long-term care is not within the mainstream of medical care.

How to provide medical care for the elderly is a controversial issue and is the subject of much discussion in Britain and the United States.[1] The United Kingdom is the only country that has developed a specialty of geriatrics.[2] Although the British Geriatric Service is considered a model for geriatric care, the future of geriatric medicine in the United Kingdom is uncertain.[3] Meanwhile, some physicians in the United States are looking to Britain for leadership and direction in the development of geriatric care.[4]

In view of this controversy, it seems therefore appropriate and useful to compare the care of the institutionalized aged in Scotland, where geriatrics is a specialty, to that in the United States, where no such specialty exists. The focus of this essay is the provision of medical care to the institutionalized aged. This is not meant to imply that medicine alone can provide health care to the elderly. The physician is one member of a team and must work collaboratively with nurses, social workers, and other paraprofessionals to plan, organize, and coordinate comprehensive care. The data presented here are part of a larger study that analyzed in detail the care of the aged in one institution in Scotland and another in the United States.[5]

Method

Data were collected during three months of fieldwork in a 96-bed, government-owned, continuing-care unit in Scotland (which I shall call "Scottsdale") and during four months of fieldwork in a similar 85-bed proprietary American nursing home (which I shall call "Pacific Manor"). A continuing-care (long-stay) unit in Scotland is comparable to a nursing home in the United States.

Selection of Institutions

Institutions comparable in size, type of patients, and services that provide medical and nursing care to aged persons with chronic, physical disabilities were selected for study. In Scotland, the government owns most health care institutions. A government institution was therefore selected as most representative. In the United States five percent of the institutions for the aged are government-owned; 18 percent are voluntary nonprofit; and 77 percent are proprietary.[6] Thus, a proprietary home, reputed to be one of the finest in the city, was selected for study in the United States.

Data Collection

Participant observation and structured interviews were used to gather data. Initially, a broad overview of life in each institution was obtained. The observer spent six to eight hours per day in the institution; observations were made at various hours throughout the day (during bathtime, mealtime, medical visits, visiting hours, and during social and recreational activities). Data were also obtained through informal interviews with physicians, nurses, therapists, and patients and their families.

A part of the study was designed to provide quantitative and qualitative data to measure patients' self-evaluation of their care. To obtain some idea of the range of opinion, 25 percent of the patients in each institution were asked a set of structured questions. Responses to the questions were ranked on a scale of 1 to 5; a 1 represented complete dissatisfaction and a 5 represented complete satisfaction with care. Subsequently, a mean was taken.

Results

Medical Care at Scottsdale

At Scottsdale, three geriatricians and one house physician provide medical care for all patients. Since the hospital consultant is a salaried employee, there is no charge to the patient for medical care. Each of the three geriatricians provides care on a continuous basis for about one-third of the patients (about 32) and visits them weekly.

In addition to the geriatrician's weekly visits, patients are seen daily by the house physician, a general practitioner on duty from 8 A.M. to 12 P.M. Monday through Friday. Although she does not visit every patient individually, she makes rounds daily, consults with the nurse in charge, and personally visits any person who needs medical attention. If a problem not within her expertise arises, she contacts the attending geriatrician. On weekends and holidays, one of the geriatricians makes rounds. Because Scottsdale is part of the geriatric service of a general hospital, the physician on call at the geriatric unit will respond if a medical emergency should arise.

Medical Care at Pacific Manor

At Pacific Manor, each patient is cared for by a private physician who charges a fee for his service. This does not mean that the elderly are responsible for all of their medical expenses. Medical care for most is paid, at least in part, by Medicare Part B (a government program for the aged) or Medicaid (a government program for the indigent). Medicare Part B, an insurance program for which the aged pay a monthly fee, does not, however, provide comprehensive coverage for all medical services. It will pay 80 percent of reasonable charges for covered services provided by physicians. Not all services are covered; for example, routine physical examinations, routine foot care, and eye or hearing examinations are not covered by Medicare.

The patients at Pacific Manor are usually visited once a month by their private physicians. Federal regulations require the physician to see a patient within 48 hours after admission and to make monthly visits thereafter. Some doctors are very conscientious and not only make the required monthly visits but come weekly or daily if the patient's condition warrants more frequent care. Not all physicians are so dutiful, however, and many patients express concern because their doctor has not visited them for several months; many feel rejected and neglected because of infrequent visits. "I called my doctor last week, but he still hasn't come," complained one woman. "He used to come when I called, but he doesn't anymore." Another woman remarked, "Some months last year my doctor didn't come at all. I told him when he came that he was falling down on the job. I don't know why he doesn't come, but I think it is because he doesn't get enough money since I am on Medicaid."

When physicians do not visit regularly, the responsibility for calling the doctor falls upon the nursing staff. Some nurses repeatedly call the physician, reminding him that he has not made the required monthly visit. If the physician does not respond, the nurse has no authority to enforce the government regulation. The regulation that patients be visited monthly appears never to have been enforced in the United States. A 1971 audit in three states disclosed that the regulation was violated in more than 50 percent of the homes surveyed.[7]

In both Scotland and the United States, the doctor is seen as the person most responsible for medical care. Thus, in order to assess satisfaction or dissatisfaction with medical care, patients were asked, "How do you find your doctor?" or "How do you feel about your medical care?"

Patients' Evaluations of Physicians' Care

At Scottsdale, the patients were highly satisfied with their medical care. In response to the above question, 80 percent of the respondents gave replies that indicated complete satisfaction with medical care, 16 percent gave an intermediate response that indicated satisfaction but not strong enthusiasm for medical care, and only one patient interviewed expressed some degree of dissatisfaction with medical care; the mean was 4.5.

At Scottsdale, responses to the question were typically very positive:

> I like my doctor very much.
> Oh, the doctors are good here; they are all good.
> My doctor is very, very nice. He usually comes twice a week.

The patients at Scottsdale were remarkably satisfied with their medical care; they felt confidence in their physician, and they knew that if they needed a doctor, one was always available.

By contrast, at Pacific Manor, the patients' responses to the same question indicated much dissatisfaction and concern about the lack of medical care. A mean of only 2.0 was obtained: 80 percent of the patients interviewed indicated dissatisfaction with their medical care; 15 percent gave an intermediate response that suggested some satisfaction with care; and 4 percent reported complete satisfaction with the medical care. At Pacific Manor, typical responses to the question, "How do you find your doctor?" ranged from neutral to negative:

> He sees me once a month. That is common, I understand, for these kinds of places.
>
> I am going to change doctors. He usually comes when I call him, but once I called him on Monday and he didn't come until Saturday. When I had the flu, he didn't come at all; he told them to give me penicillin, and I am allergic to penicillin.
>
> They are supposed to come once a month, but sometimes my doctor skips. I don't think he likes to come here.

Many of the elderly expressed concern about lack of attention to medical needs. Patients seemed to realize, however, that they were entitled to only one visit per month. The limitation of a monthly medical visit produced apprehension in the elderly ("I could die before my doctor came again.") and made it difficult for the nursing staff to request additional visits.

This problem is poignantly illustrated in the case of Mrs. L., a 73-year-old woman with terminal cancer. Since Mrs. L.'s admission to the nursing home on January 12, 1978, the nurse had repeatedly called the doctor asking him to see her; however, although the law says he must visit within 48 hours after admission, he did not come until January 19, 1978. Two weeks later on February 3, 1978, Mrs. L.'s cousin (her only relative) asked the nurse to call the doctor and request a visit. The nurse called the doctor, explained that the family was concerned, that the patient's condition appeared terminal, and asked if he could make a visit. The doctor replied that he only had to visit once a month, that he did not have time to come to the nursing home, and that if the family were dissatisfied, they could get another doctor. Both the nurse and the patient's relative were very upset. Later, the nurse said: "We know there is nothing he can do medically; all we are asking for is a little humanitarianism, but he has none to give. I get this all the time with doctors who have patients in the nursing home; they admit them and just write them off."

Other staff and patients made similar statements suggesting that patients at Pacific Manor feel—and probably are—neglected by their physicians. One nurse remarked that on some occasions when she had suggested glasses or a hearing aid for a patient, the doctor had declined the suggestion with, "Oh well, she's old anyhow," and a patient observed, "There are too many people here whom the doctors have rejected or turned away." A speech therapist who periodically came to the nursing home put it succinctly: "I would rather work in an acute-care hospital. The patients in nursing homes are the ones the doctors have given up on."

On one occasion, a physician admitted an elderly woman to the nursing home and then refused to care for her. Eighty-nine year old Mrs. E. had been in an acute care hospital with a fractured hip. "When he told me I had to leave the hospital, he said he would come here to see me," she explained. "He was my doctor for 15 years; now they say he has released me to a new doctor, whom I do not even know." When Mrs. E.'s physician refused to care for her in the nursing home, the nurses had to locate another doctor to write admission orders. Thinking there must be some misunderstanding, I approached Mrs. E.'s newly acquired physician and asked what had happened to her personal physician. "He just abandoned her," he said.

Clearly, there is wide variation both in the quantity and quality of medical care in the two institutions. At Scottsdale, the adequacy of medical care was never a subject for discussion. Indeed, it was simply understood that patients would receive whatever medical care was necessary. At Pacific Manor, however, the lack of medical care was frequently a subject for discussion with patients, their families, and nursing staff.

Discussion

The overall purpose of this research was to investigate criteria for quality of care and to attempt to discover what institutional structures encourage the maintenance of high standards of care. The results of this study provide evidence that at Scottsdale the geriatrician is a catalyst in promoting quality care whereas at Pacific Manor, in general, the physician did little to promote high standards of care.

The outstanding medical care at Scottsdale cannot be attributed solely to the presence of geriatricians. Providing long-term care to the elderly is a complex issue that involves historical, social, cultural, political, and economic factors. In comparing the medical care of the aged in these two institutions, however, certain structural and philosophical differences were observed.

At Scottsdale, the geriatric service provided a structure for the provision of acute and long-term care for the elderly. Within the structure, the geriatrician, utilizing a multidisciplinary team approach, emphasized continuity of care. The attitude of the health team was one of hope, of maximizing the independence of the aged, and of providing them with all necessary services, both medical and social. The geriatrician not only provided leadership, he set the standards and took the responsibility for overseeing continuing, comprehensive care of the aged. The weekly visit of the geriatricians demonstrated their steadfast involvement even after the acute phase of illness had subsided. The patients' satisfaction with medical care illustrates that the geriatrician (a specialist with clinical expertise) had appropriately assessed their needs, provided optimal medical care, and continued to be concerned with their care. Patients commented that everything possible was being done for them, and they contentedly accepted Scottsdale as their homes for the rest of their lives.

By comparison, at Pacific Manor there was no structure to ensure adequate, continuing medical care (care was often custodial) and there was no evidence of a team approach to care. The behavior of the physicians conveyed an attitude of lack of concern and hopelessness as expressed by the speech therapist who said: "The patients in the nursing homes are the ones the doctors have given up on." The physicians at Pacific Manor did not provide leadership, or take the responsibility for medical care, and in some cases there was a complete abdication of responsibility for care. This abdication of responsibility by the physician caused anxiety and fear among patients and created frustration among the nursing staff who were powerless to ameliorate the situation.

The infrequent and perfunctory visits of physicians further illustrate a lack of interest in the responsibility for the medical care of the aged. Ingman,[8] in a questionnaire survey, found a relatively strong consensus among nurses, physicians, and nursing home administrators to the statement: "Lack of physician interest in geriatric medicine is a major problem in long-term care."[9] The lack of physician responsibility for patient care at Pacific Manor, undoubtedly, is related to the philosophy of medical care in the United States. Traditionally, the emphasis in American medicine has been on acute care. The rewards, both financial and professional, are greater in treating acute illness, and physicians have not been trained to deal with the unique problems of aging.[10] Yet many of the medical problems of old age are chronic in nature, and chronic conditions are especially prevalent among elderly residents of nursing homes.[11]

Although British medicine has traditionally also given a higher priority to acute illness than to chronic disability,[12] a group of concerned and dedicated physicians have succeeded in establishing geriatrics as a specialty, providing outstanding leadership in geriatric care. [13] It is unlikely that the high quality of medical care at Scottsdale would have been possible without this leadership and expertise. Wright notes that geriatricians who devoted themselves wholly to the specialty were responsible for considerable progress in the care of the elderly. In discussing the future development of geriatric medicine in Britain, he remarks that only physicians who are completely committed to the sick elderly are able to give them the comprehensive care they deserve. Furthermore, he concludes that geriatrics must continue to exist as a specialty in order to maintain satisfactory standards for medical care of the aged.[14] Yet, as mentioned earlier, the future of geriatric medicine is uncertain in the United Kingdom, and the development of geriatrics as a specialty in the United States seems dubious at this time. Recently, a committee of the Institute of Medicine of the National Academy of Sciences recommended against the development of a board-certified specialty of geriatrics. The committee noted that "most problems of the elderly do not require the services of geriatricians," and that "the care of the aged should continue to be the responsibility of well-trained primary care physicians."[15]

In the United States, physicians in internal medicine, family practice, and psychiatry provide the bulk of medical care to the aged.

Carboni discusses the diffusion of responsibility that occurs when geriatric medicine is theoretically included in many medical specialties but is claimed exclusively by none. On the other hand, the development of a medical specialty has a number of positive consequences. It provides an identity for those interested in the area, and provides leaders in the specialty who can compete for resources, promote research, and organize as an advocacy group to lobby for the special interests of those being served by the specialty.[16]

Since the inception of the National Health Service, British geriatricians have made tremendous progress in developing a system of patient care to treat the multiple, complex sociomedical problems of old age. Prior to that time, physicians had been referring the elderly with chronic problems to geriatric hospitals. These hospitals, understaffed, underequipped, and out of reach of medical attention, were used for the disposal of clinical failures.[17]

In the U.S., where geriatrics is not yet a specialty, there is an absence of physician involvement in long-term care of the elderly; the care is fragmented, often custodial in nature, and the nursing home has become a place of last resort for those elderly patients who cannot remain in acute institutions, and who are unable to manage in the community. The nursing home stands as a symbol of the inadequacy of the health system to meet the needs of the aged.[18]

The comparison of the medical care of the elderly in these two institutions suggests that the nursing home in the United States in the 1970s is similar in many respects to the geriatric hospital in the United Kingdom in the early 1940s. In discussing the future of geriatrics as a specialty in Britain, it has been suggested that 1) the specialty be abandoned; 2) it be an age-related specialty such as pediatrics; and 3) geriatrics be integrated with the rest of medicine while preserving what has previously been achieved.[19] Perhaps before choosing any of these options, British physicians should examine the current situation of geriatric care in the United States and consider the following: 1) the progress and status that British geriatrics has achieved despite political and economic problems; 2) the benefits that geriatricians have provided to the elderly; and 3) what the future consequences would be for the chronically disabled elderly if the present system were altered or abandoned.

The findings of this research provide evidence that serious problems exist in providing medical care to nursing home residents in the United States. Scottsdale provides an excellent model for long-term care; the data suggest that the elderly are highly satisfied with their care. The role of the geriatrician is so central to the quality of care that it is difficult to imagine that the welfare of the nursing home patient will improve without the development of geriatrics as a specialty in the United States. Nursing can be influential in raising the standards of care, but without the support and cooperation of knowledgeable physicians, progress may be slow. Nursing home residents require a full range of medical, psychological, and social services, yet American physicians are trained almost exclusively in acute care hospitals, have little experience in planning and implementing long-term care, and are exposed to little if any geriatric training in medical school curricula.

Providing long-term care to the elderly has been and will continue to be a problem of considerable magnitude in the United Kingdom and the United States. The Scottish experience demonstrates that maximum benefits can be achieved when professionals skilled and knowledgeable in geriatrics work together in a team fashion to provide continuing, comprehensive care for the elderly. The development of geriatrics as a specialty in the United Kingdom is clearly a positive approach that addresses the health needs of the aged, and the United States can learn a great deal from the British experience. In both countries, it is critical that future planning and decision making be based on society's needs rather than on conflicts within the profession. Physicians in both countries may encounter political struggles in their attempt to compete for resources and to design and maintain programs for long-term care of the aged. Their success or failure will largely determine the quality of care for the aged in future years.

Notes

[1]F. Anderson, "Geriatric Medicine: An Academic Discipline," *Age and Aging* 5 (1976):193.

Butler, R. N. *Why Survive? Being Old in America* (St. Louis: The C. V. Mosby Company, 1975).

Clarke, S. C., J. Badenock, and D. A. Winner, et al., "Medical Care of The Elderly," *Lancet* 1 (1977):1092.

Exton-Smith, A. N., and J. G. Evans (eds.), *Care of the Elderly: Meeting the Challenge of Dependency* (New York: Grune 1977).

Leonard, J. C. "Can Geriatrics Survive?" *Br. Med. Journal* 1 (1977):1335.

Reichel, W. (ed.), "Proceedings of the American Geriatrics Society Conferences on Geriatric Education," *J. of American Geriatrics Society* 55 (1977):481.

Rossman, I. "Why We Shy Away from Geriatrics," *Geriatrics* 36, July (1976).

Somers, A. R. "Geriatric Care in the United Kingdom: An American Perspective," *American Journal of Int. Medicine* 84 (1976):466.

Williamson, J. "Notes on the Historical Development of Geriatric Medicine as a Specialty," *Age and Aging* 8 (1979):144.

Wilson, L. A. "Geriatrics at the Crossroads," *Geront. Clin.* 14 (1972):193.

Wright, W. B. "Geriatrics and General Medicine," *Age and Aging* 1 (1972):120.

[2]J. Williamson, "Notes on the Historical Development."

[3]R. W. Stout, "Three Views on Geriatric Medicine: Hospital Care of the Elderly: General or Geriatric Medicine?" *Age and Aging* 8 (1979):137.

[4]W. R. Hazzard, "Three Views on Geriatric Medicine: An American's Ode to British Geriatrics," *Age and Aging* 8 (1979):141.

[5]J. S. Kayser-Jones, *Old, Alone and Neglected: Care of the Aged in Scotland and the United States* (Berkeley, CA. and London: University of California Press, 1981).

[6]U. S. Department of Health, Education, and Welfare (1979), *The National Nursing Home Survey: 1977 Summary for the United States*. Washington, D.C.: U. S. Government Printing Office.

[7]F. E. Moss, and V. J. Halamandaris, *Too Old, Too Sick, Too Bad: Nursing Homes in America* (Aspen Systems Corp., Rockville, MD, 1977).

[8]S. R. Ingman, I. R. Lawson, and D. Carboni, "Medical Direction in Long-Term Care," *J. of the American Geriatrics Society* 26 (1978):157.

[9]U. S. Senate Special Committee on Aging Subcommittee on Long-Term Care: *Nursing Home Care in the U. S.: Failure in Public Policy. Supporting paper No. 3: Doctors in Nursing Homes—The Shunned Responsibility*. Washington, D.C.: U. S. Government Printing Office, 1975.

[10]R. N. Butler, *Why Survive?*

[11]M. G. Kovar, Testimony Before the Select Committee and the Select Committee on Population. U. S. House of Representatives, 1978.

[12]R. W. Stout, "Three Views."

[13]G. F. Adams, "Origins and Destiny of British Geriatrics," *Age and Aging* 4 (1975):65.

[14]W. B. Wright, "Geriatrics and General Medicine."

[15]P. J. Dans, and M. R. Kerr, "Gerontology and Geriatrics in Medical Education," *The New England Journal of Medicine* 300 (1979):228.

[16]D. K. Carboni, "Geriatrics: To Be or Not to Be a Medical Specialty," *Sociological Symposium*, Vol. 19 (1977), pp. 104–115.

[17]D. K. Carboni, "To Be or Not To Be."

[18]R. L. Kane, & R. A. Kane, "Care of the Aged: Old Problems in Need of New Solutions," *Science*, 200(1978):913.

[19]J. Williamson, "Notes on the Historical Development."

PART II
TEACHING GERIATRIC MEDICAL CARE

6
Humanistic Geriatric Care: A Context of Antitheses

IAN R. LAWSON

Introduction

Our society, its demographic momentum, and its yield of aged persons are the product of living standards the like of which have never been seen before. These high standards are, unfortunately, now confined to our region of the world—the "West and North"—and (in line with the projections of "Global 2000") probably will not extend beyond it. Excepting nuclear war, this demographic momentum will continue to effect population changes into the last two decades of this millennium and the first three or four decades of the next. Most of us alive now will participate in it. Indeed, we shall all become a part of its chief and most numerous result, for we shall survive and grow old, and many of us will grow old and dependent. Around 2000 A.D., when many of us become members of those decades of dependency, there will be twice as many of us in our 70s and 80s as there are now.

The personal consequences of being old can be profoundly upsetting in both their unexpectedness and their effects on daily life. They are more so when one has lived in a society that, more than any other, has organized itself around the ideal of personal autonomy, mastery of the environment, and the notion of a future with perpetual options. A lady in her late 60s, having recently lost her second husband and now immobilized by a cast for a fractured leg, said to me: "I've always been a forward-looking person and I'm having to adjust to not having a future to look forward to." What she meant was that there was a future, but it was altogether less promising of relationship and options than the remembered past. There had occurred not only a radical turn of events but of prospects. She had suffered a loss both of relationship and of future. This experience is discordant with the culture of which she is a part, with her own habituation to it, and with the social systems that have been constructed to support her typical ideals and notions.

Those who make their vocation the medical care of dependent elderly may therefore find the going more rugged than their well-intentioned natures would have anticipated. The medical profession at large, American society, and even the elderly constituency had other scenarios in mind. Though compassionate, practical, and skillful—welcome indeed to those who have met their nemesis in the pathologies of aging—geriatric medicine still must address a reality which is offensive and unwelcome, not to the young who are too remote to sense it, but to the middle-aged and younger elderly whose social and professional consensus is determinative of what is done or not done in social organization. Therefore, the antitheses to be described are rational at one level only. That they also originate from the emotions and ambivalence of the middle-aged consensus may explain why the dysfunctional cybernetics of our present social organization persist as they do. The common rationalization that America is a "youth-oriented society" is a further symptom of a denial syndrome—an arrogation to youth of faults that the middle-age sector sees in itself.

Probably no subject in the curriculum is as dependent for its final effect upon the humanity of the milieu in which it is preached and practiced as is geriatrics. While the proliferation of courses on geriatrics run by medical schools would imply that geriatrics is merely a matter of knowledge content and of emphasizing certain chronologic effects upon organ systems, their diseases and treatments, geriatric medicine is, in fact, a demonstrably different way of practice with respect to distressed dependent, elderly people. There is a palpable and self-communicating ethos required. That is, there is a recognizable genius or spirit in those institutions, agencies, and groups which practice geriatrics as an avocation. There is a good deal of ethical debate and soul-searching as to what is right and wise in patient care. How to achieve it, that is, the processes of care, are the means rather than the end of care. Independence in the activities of daily functioning, relationship to family and environment, self-image and self-worth are given enormous attention in a detail that fast-track hospital systems generally treat as peripheral.

Geriatric medicine is an enjoyable pursuit confined, for the most part, to those who practice the kind of detailed, considerate, painstaking work that effective care of the elderly requires. This enjoyment is important since it contributes not only to the ethos of the patient care team but also to a necessary self-sufficiency of motivation and satisfaction; for geriatric practice must survive a context of systems and professional regard in the United States that is still persistently antithetical. The reasons for this situation are manifold and mutually reinforcing.

First, there are differences of nosographic emphases that imply a fundamental difference of perspective on patient experience. Geriatrics focuses on distress and disability more than on extension of elderly life. Hence, symptoms are not merely clues that lead the medical problem solver to those peer criteria we call diagnostic answers. Symptoms are suffering; they are part of the experience of elderly distress. The other parts of that experience which have, to date, barely made it into medical nosography, are: unaccustomed restrictions of the activities and options of daily life; a dependency on and vulnerability towards a physical environment over which one was once master; a dependency relationship with significant others that compels their giving (and one's own receiving) on mutually inconvenient terms of neither's making; and the loss of a materially hopeful future.

Even palliative activities towards these distresses require a medical practice of broad and exacting scope. Moreover, when the anatomic and physiologic factors are unmalleable, geriatrics must then attempt a reconstruction of the ecology of dependency. Engineering of institutional structure and function to yield the prosthetic milieu is required. The same is true for the home. Some modification may be required in the psychodynamics of the natural relationships of dependency—relationships with sons, daughters, spouse, or neighbors. Even the personality functioning of professional and care-providing staff must be recruited and disciplined to provide prosthetic and surrogate relationships.

These sets of care-providing functions and engineering functions themselves depend, first, on exquisite clinical and observational skills, and second, on an appropriate biology—an accurate conception and factual reference in regard to what illness and disability is about in the very elderly. The difficulties in teaching these functions are not solely due to the multiple morbidities of the burdened elderly; nor are they due to some imagined incompatibility between them and young trainees. The problems of teaching geriatrics occur with those of practicing it in antithetical contexts: they are professional, fiscal, administrative, and academic. The nature of the antitheses must be understood in order to make these contexts at least partially usable. For all their dysfunctional cybernetics and countercurrents, they are the only supporting contexts we presently have. However, "making do" with them and educating our trainees in the ethical exploitation of them on behalf of patient care should not absolve faculty of the duty to advocate change.

Antitheses

Antitheses in the medical professional context arise from the "acute" and "curative" notions in medical care, from the momentum of high technology hospital processes and from the favored predominance of medical subspecialism in continuing medical education, hospital process, and the financial-rewards system. I like to describe this doctor-hospital complex as a "black hole" phenomenon—so massive and compact that it pulls in the resources for even modest alternatives to the further accrual of its own density! Like the other contexts, it is essential, as well as essentially faulty. It is at its best in elective care of selected problems of the infirm elderly; it is at its worst in terminal, intensive care of multiple system failure where it seems compelled more by process rather than chosen for benefits. Antitheses in the fiscal context exists in the way medical care for the elderly is paid for by the public systems of support under title 18 (Medicare) and title 19 (Medicaid) enactments. Designed around the preferred incentives of providers rather than around the characteristics of elderly need, they have propagated and powerfully reinforced, rather than modified, the antitheses of the professional context. Antitheses in the administrative context, especially institutional, arise from the conditions of operation set by the fiscal context. Even in nonprofit institutions, programs are sponsored according to their ability to fill beds and capture "third party" eligibility and funding status. Institutional administrators are required to oversee the minutiae of care because their itemization determines, under fee for service, the remuneration of the institution and the administrator's "bottom line" success or failure. Hence, propagating individualized, imaginative actions of care may be countercurrent to the institutional systems of control and finance. Effective, interdisciplinary teamwork can be particularly irritating because of the functional autonomy and group ethos necessary to sustain it. Hence, some sense of alienation is universally felt by case workers toward the institutions of which they are a part and toward the public systems in which they must function. This appears to be a notable American phenomenon. This sense, however, needs to be disciplined and sublimated in order for the client to get optimal—although not ideal—care, for preserving the institution in its working imperfection and for the case professional to be spared from "burnout."

The antitheses between geriatric care and academia exist, first, by virtue of the present organization of academia in tension with the needed professionalism of geriatric medicine. In regard to clinical specialism, academia confers identity according to single organ system interest or high technology pursuits. Geriatric medicine, on the contrary, is a study of interactive pathologies and of these with treatments and environment; its technology is the "software" of communication and delivery systems in multiple phases of care; its practices are those of elective parsimony, acting modestly and earlier in preference to emergently, and "acutely" later. Intellectually, as well as operationally, this kind of holism is very difficult to sustain. Even family practice (imploded into academia by a vigorous guild advocacy from without) emerges as an uneasy and ambivalent supporter of geriatrics, whose practices are frequently too intense and detailed and whose large scale requirements are too prominent to be supported within the declared nonspecialism of the former. The Institute of Medicine's recommendation, therefore, that geriatrics should have curricular place but not specialty practice status appears to result from a negative consensus of established medical interest rather than as a positive advocacy from within the field.

In addition, geriatrics' working holism of care appears to academics as merely a pragmatic composite of what every good specialist should know about his or her particular bit of the elderly body. While European history indicates that clinical scientific interest in the elderly emerged primarily from its specialty practice, geriatric medicine in the United States is not currently regarded as capable of sustaining original research or theory except for those of its practitioners who emerge with conventional subspecialty alliances. The elderly body is viewed as a field of divisible interests, notwithstanding the demonstrable fact that the practice of geriatric care depends on an integrated management of systems interactions.

A third reason for the antithesis between geriatrics and medical academia is the notion of what is opportune therapeutically, that is, the manipulable stuff of medical care of the elderly patients. High technology subspecialism in internal medicine supports intensive, focal investigation in order to obtain either a molecular, physiologic, or anatomical characterization of the elderly person's disorder. It may be pursued so vigorously as to threaten the total organism's well-being and viability, and it can result in a plethora of data of such unmanageable size and confusion that critically relevant signals are lost. It commonly neglects altogether the ecology of dependency, regarding it as a nonmedical area, even when it contributes unique pathophysiologic and iatrogenic insights.

The reasons for such selective and intense pursuits lie in premises about how and where leverage for beneficial change may be applied in patient care. Empirically, practitioners of geriatric care find that a focal intensity of investigation of patients may have less utility than a broader span of attention, which includes—as emphasized earlier—recognition of contributory problems from other systems as well as interactions with the environment. Then there is also this matter of critical parsimony of diagnostic and therapeutic effort.

This parsimony is conducted out of respect to the fragile physiology of the patient and because the goals of care are primarily those of improving function and symptoms. "Cure" of "disease" is applicable to only a minority of situations. Applied to the very elderly patient, this parsimony will restrict the intensity and the number of diagnostic and therapeutic elements. The goals of functional restoration and mental well-being are as targeted and as elaborately described as the use of laboratory and drugs are restrained. In the hospital environment, astir intellectually with the notion that power is knowing more, geriatrics is a counterargument for finding out less but knowing more relevantly. Those who practice and argue for it within such environments expect adversarial confrontations with teachers and their trainees as a matter of course, but the crippling lack of alternative models may deny this counterargument the empiric substantiation that is needed for lasting didactic effect.

Hence the ultimate and personal antithesis in geriatric medicine is what the doctor practicing it thought he was going to do and be, especially in reference to the body politic of medicine, and how he now appears to himself in his developed role towards the dependent elderly. At a meeting of the New York Medical Directors Association a year ago, its president, Jack Muth, M.D., listed three ingredients that discourage physician involvement in even a modest leadership role in the nursing home. First, there was the severe disability of many nursing home residents, much of it intractable. Second, there was the ever-present disregard of elderly care by medical colleagues. Third, there was oppressive regulation, as inhibiting to the good as it was intended to be to the bad. What answer can physicians give to themselves, not to mention to the public, for their continued involvement in such a field? I could only answer "authentic concern" which leads me back to my opening dictum—the need for self-sustenance.

Nationally, the case and care of the dependent elderly, both homebound and resident in institutions, is an index of progression or regression of the apparatus and ethos of medical care and, cybernetically, is a paradigm of what is effective or dysfunctional about societal and institutional systems at large. Historically, it is a product of social and demographic momenta having a continuing and accelerating effect. It will not go away. Herein lies another antithetical context, that is, the sobering prospect from geriatric medicine of a growing number of dependent elderly requiring care in tension with the futurism of a facile gerontology. The idea is that we may be able so to reconstruct ourselves biomedically that the end of life will be an immediate and total dissolution, sparing ourselves and others the tedium of end-of-life dependency. Even in nonagenarians no such form of death has as yet been recorded. It is Holmes's whimsy of the "one hoss shay"* adopted for the marketing of biomedical enterprises. This image of instantaneous disolution is a mere abstraction, not sustained at autopsy.

Concluding Word

Elderly dependency is one of the principal phenomena of our society, and an inescapable experience through which, short of nuclear catastrophe, most of us alive now will pass. The scale, complexity, and enterprise it requires of medicine is dependent on a metanoia of both medical and political minds of an order and direction that seems presently unlikely. Our culture may in the end be rendered impotent by the unstable coalition of its constituents. We may be unable to function in the organized manner necessary to cope with these human consequences of demography and unsurpassed living standards. We may continue to be driven by popular ideologies derived from never-again times of plethora, ideologies that support only the most direct and rudimentary of market reward systems: "Me first, for the most, now"—a modern barbarism cloaked, however, by ingenious apologetics and economics.

*A literary analogy comparing the human body with a horse-drawn cart built to last a prearranged finite time and then instantaneously dissolve.

In more than one sense, therefore, geriatric medicine is the discipline of providing effective, uplifting personal care (and systems of care) within a human and societal future that is ominous. Not one of us so involved would doubt the worth of the endeavor, a sense of worth that derives in large part from the therapeutic as well as personal responsiveness of those time-limited, life-as-lived people we call "elderly." Surely these positive transactions of giving and receiving, set as they are within the ambivalences of the larger context, are redolent of opportunities for the humanities. Their involvement in concert with medical care need not be justified on utilitarian grounds of doing things better. But, in fact, because these contributions challenge and enrich the perspectives and insights of those providing care, they can also contribute to the ecosystems of care we construct around elderly dependency. There is, for instance, no more critical issue in geriatric care than how we can support elderly self-respect and morale or subvert them both, using the same instruments and institutions of care. In order to practice the one as opposed to the other, determinative professionals need to know the difference exquisitely: if their sensitivities are to be enhanced by professional humanists, they also have to be present at and see the real interfaces of geriatric care. Long-term institutional care is incredibly more complicated than even academic clinicians recognize; it is often more kindly and well-meaning than the publicized scandals would imply; and it is equipped with more insights and skills towards its dilemmas of care than the scholarly but aloof is often aware of.

7

Medical Student Education In Teaching Nursing Homes

FREDRICK T. SHERMAN

Introduction

A range of opinion, significant academic experiences, and a growing body of research support the concept that teaching nursing homes should be settings for training medical students in geriatric medicine.[1] A comprehensive program, based in one or more nursing homes, and having rehabilitative, long-term, ambulatory, and home care components, would provide the educational forum for teaching geriatrics. Elderly people residing in such a nursing home, either temporarily or permanently, and the frail, community-residing elderly, would use these services. Each medical school should affiliate with a large multilevel long-term care institution or a number of smaller institutions in order to develop comprehensive clinical, educational, and research programs in geriatrics.

This essay will discuss the special knowledge, approaches, and skills needed to deal with the multiple medical, psychiatric, rehabilitative, and social problems of the institutionalized and "near-institutionalized" elderly. It will also describe previous nursing home-based, geriatric medical programs, and present a plan for the progressive four-year involvement of medical students in a prototypic geriatric medical program. An educational program led by physi-

Presented, in part, at an American College of Physicians' Conference: The Changing Needs of Nursing Home Care, Washington, D.C.

cians who are trained as academic geriatricians and are knowledgeable about organizing and delivering health care services to the
elderly would be the medical school faculty, based partially or totally
in such academic nursing homes.

Medical Student Training in Nursing Homes and Other Long-term Care Institutions

Need

If the physicians of the future are to intelligently manage the growing number of disabled older people, they must have educational and
training experiences in the long-term care phases of health and
illness in the elderly. Current practice patterns reveal that general
physicians are extensively involved in nursing home care. In a 1982
survey of general physicians in Missouri, over 50 percent routinely
attended to patients in nursing homes, with approximately one-fifth
serving as medical directors.[2] One-third to one-half of all patients on
general medical services at acute general teaching hospitals are over
the age of 65. Large numbers of these older patients in acute hospitals
have disabilities that are strikingly comparable, in type and degree,
to those found in nursing home patients.[3] Approximately five percent of acute hospital beds in a major metropolitan area is used by
elderly patients awaiting nursing home placement. Because the
acute hospital environment is not ideally suited to the teaching of
geriatric medicine on patients with advanced levels of disability,
nursing home teaching programs are necessary. With the growing
number of old people over age 75, the number of dependent elderly people in nursing homes, acute hospitals, and the community
will increase.[4]

Current Status

Medical and governmental organizations that have assessed the need
for medical student education in clinical gerontology and geriatric
medicine have recommended that nursing homes and other long-
term care institutions be used as training sites.[5] The Institute of
Medicine, for example, in its report, *Aging and Medical Education*
(September 1978), recommends that "nursing homes and other long-

term care facilities be included in clinical rotations for medical students and housestaff." In 1974, 74 percent of all medical schools that replied to a questionnaire from the U.S. Senate Special Committee on Aging claimed they had "a program whereby students and interns could work in nursing homes."[6] Two years later, only 40 percent of the medical schools that replied continued to have such programs, indicating an unexplained decline in medical student training in nursing homes. The vast majority of these programs were and continue to be elective.

The Association of American Medical Colleges' 1979–1980 Curriculum Directory lists 73 of 125 medical schools (58 percent) as having elective opportunities in geriatrics.[7] The directory does not, however, specify whether any portion of the elective is given in a nursing home. A review of the American Medical Student Association's *Clinical Geriatrics Training Site Directory* reveals that of 63 medical schools that describe geriatric electives available to medical students, only 34 involve a nursing home as a site in which teaching took place.[8] Twelve of these 34 electives (35 percent) were exclusively based in nursing homes and were only available to third and fourth year students. The programs were directed by departments of medicine, family practice, community and preventive medicine, or rehabilitation medicine. Many of the elective programs that exposed students to clinical gerontology and geriatric medicine during the first and second years used the nursing home as one of many sites for education and training.

Previous Program Initiatives

M. Rodstein, chairman of the Committee on Undergraduate and Continuing Medical Education of the Clinical Medicine Section of the Gerontological Society of America, described a three-week, full-time clinical elective in clinical gerontology and geriatric medicine for medical students based in a long-term care institution.[9] The elective included both clinical and didactic components. The clinical aspect emphasized techniques for interviewing the elderly, physical diagnosis, case presentations, medical and geropsychiatric rounds, as well as observation and participation in medical, general surgery, psychiatry, rehabilitation, and peripheral vascular disease clinics. Didactic information about the aged, presented in seminars and readings, included the following areas with specific geriatric emphasis: orthopedics, pathology, radiology, cardiology, surgery, accidents and accident prevention, arthritis, gastrointestinal disease, hematological, urological, and gynecological problems, and pharmacy and therapeutics. Students were also introduced to the principles of rehabilitation medicine, occupational and physical therapy, reality orientation, sheltered workshops, social service, senior citizen centers, the day hospital, and research methodology. The Committee concluded that the organization and supervision of such a course would take a considerable commitment by highly interested faculty members based in the long-term care institution.

Although the number of programs in which medical students have clinical experiences in nursing homes is increasing, only one required program has been well-studied from an attitudinal viewpoint.[10] In that program, students in a mandatory family practice clerkship spent four or five half-day sessions learning about gerontology and geriatrics in a 260-bed proprietary nursing home under the tutelage of a family practice faculty member and a chief resident. The students were given one-hour didactic sessions on each of the following topics: physiology of senescence, common clinical problems associated with old age, prescribing for the elderly, psychosocial issues of institutionalized and home care patients, and community resources available to serve the aged.

Subsequently, visits were made to assigned patients who they examined and followed clinically for the entire five-week period. The patients were chronically ill and usually disoriented. Student attitudes toward the elderly, while improving during this nursing home rotation, did not improve as much as the attitudes of students who had an elective entitled "Understanding and Caring for the Elderly," that empathetically focused on healthy, active, community-residing elderly. Attitudes toward the rehabilitation potential of the elderly improved in this community-based elective experience but remained unchanged in the required nursing home clerkship. Students voiced uneasiness about spending four half-days in a nursing home with large numbers of confused patients. They also felt uncertain about their medical role with chronically disabled patients. Subsequently, the faculty modified the clerkship to provide more experience with community-residing elderly people.

Somers has reported a similar experience in a second-year family medicine elective in geriatrics, based predominantly in a 300-bed chronic disease institution.[11] The curriculum included 11 three-hour sessions. Each session consisted of a one-hour didactic component, a one-hour interview with a chronically ill elderly patient and his or her family (as well as health care providers) and a final hour of clinical rounds on patients with medical, psychiatric, and social problems. Other sessions emphasized home care, discharge planning, death and dying, and socioeconomic problems of the elderly. Student assessment of the course was varied. Many remarked about their difficulty communicating with deaf, depressed, or demented patients. The authors commented on the problems they faced in developing a long-term care experience for the entire medical school class, because of the lack of an affiliated institution having a well-developed program in which faculty had a major commitment to teaching geriatrics. Based on the students' initial experiences, an elective with a more balanced view of geriatric practice was recommended, including sessions at a day care center and a housing development for the elderly, as well as in the chronic disease institution.

A summer program in gerontology and geriatric medicine at the New York University School of Medicine has been developed for first- and second-year medical students, which emphasizes the health care needs of the elderly, the development of positive attitudes toward working with the elderly, and the need for a multidisciplinary approach to their problems.[12] The program consists of field placements (many of which are in nursing homes), a seminar series, and an interpersonal skills laboratory program that emphasizes geriatric interviewing skills. A physician who is a positive role model for geriatrics is selected as a preceptor in the field placement. This program has grown to include 50 students from all over the country.

A model elective, clinical clerkship for third- and fourth-year medical students has been developed at the Jewish Institute for Geriatric Care, a 527-bed skilled nursing institution, that is academically affiliated and physically connected with the Long Island Jewish–Hillside Medical Center, a teaching campus of the Health Sciences Center of the State University of New York at Stony Brook. The four-to-six-week clerkship consists of clinical encounters during the acute, rehabilitative, chronic, and home care phases of treatment as well as didactic experiences. A modular curriculum for medical students has been developed based on these experiences.[13] Students transfering to U.S. internships from foreign medical schools, physician's assistant students, and geriatric nurse practitioner students have also rotated through the program as part of a requirement of their respective training programs.

Williams has described an elective clinical clerkship based at the Monroe Community Hospital, a 938-bed chronic disease institution that is academically affiliated with the University of Rochester

School of Medicine and Dentistry. This elective includes many of the previously described components.[14]

In general, there appears to be a positive attitudinal response to experiences based partially or totally in nursing homes. When a brief mandatory or elective geriatric course takes place only at a nursing home, attitudes improve—but not as much as in programs exposing students to elderly who reside both in the community and in the institution. Geriatric programs for first- and second-year students involving field placements at nursing homes—supplemented with didactic and interviewing sessions—have been successful. Finally, third- and fourth-year elective clerkships and required rotations for fifth pathway students, are well received when the programs cover the acute, rehabilitative, long-term, and home care phases of illness as taught by positively motivated physicians trained in geriatrics.

If we are to proceed further with the expectation of developing and integrating nursing home experiences into medical student education, we must answer the following basic questions: 1) What aspects of clinical gerontology and geriatrics are appropriately taught in the nursing home? 2) What specific attitudes, concepts, and approaches should be demonstrated and taught, and how will these be integrated into a comprehensive program in clinical gerontology and geriatrics? 3) Who will do the teaching? 4) How will the educational programs in nursing homes be supported and evaluated?

The Use of the Nursing Home in Geriatric Medical Education

While the medical student will see and care for many acutely ill geriatric patients during his or her training (30 to 50 percent of patients on acute medical and surgical wards are over age 65), the student may not learn geriatric medicine. In the nursing home, where the average patient's age is 82, the effect of age on presentation, diagnosis, and therapy of multiple illnesses and disabilities must be addressed. The differentiation between normal aging, disease, and disability must be emphasized if rational therapy is to be prescribed.

In the nursing home the student will see the results of chronic physical and mental illness in the elderly and develop an approach to assessment and treatment not usually stressed in other health care settings.[15] Patients will present a wide variety of chronic illnesses and disabilities, as well as a limited number of acute and subacute problems, including diseases or syndromes seen almost exclusively in the elderly (e.g., fractured hip, senile dementia of the Alzheimer's type (SDAT), recurrent falls, cerebrovascular accidents, urinary incontinence, asymptomatic bacteriuria, systolic hypertension, and prostatic hypertrophy) as well as diseases occurring in all adult ages but with different presentation, pathophysiology, or appropriate treatment in the elderly (e.g., myocardial infarction, hyperglycemia, diastolic hypertension, anemia, and depression). The acute presentation of these problems is usually seen in the hospital where rapid diagnosis and treatment by the traditional medical and surgical approaches are taught.

Nursing home patients in the subacute, recovery, and chronic maintenance phases of illness require approaches and skills unique to geriatric medicine. For example, the diagnosis and stabilization of the elderly patient with an acute cerebrovascular accident is usually taught in the hospital. The skilled nursing setting, however, is the most likely place to teach the approach to the rehabilitation phase of stroke and the effect that multiple acute and chronic illnesses can have on stroke recovery in the elderly patient. Similarly, the management of the medically and psychiatrically complex elderly patient recovering from a fractured hip or amputation, or being treated for chronic congestive heart failure, cancer, dementia, or any combination of these, is best illustrated in the nursing home. Impaired mobility, falls, and urinary and/or fecal incontinence are frequently seen in nursing home patients.[16] The diagnosis and treatment of these potentially reversible, yet often neglected disorders, are aptly highlighted in this setting.[17]

The principles of physical medicine and rehabilitation that apply to the geriatric patient can be taught to medical students by the physiatrist and geriatrician with the assistance of physical and occupational therapists. The rehabilitative approach to elderly patients with a fractured hip, stroke, amputation, arthritis, or disuse and impaired ambulation from multiple causes, can also be best taught in the skilled nursing setting. The student can observe an "activities of daily living" (ADL) evaluation and learn about practical devices that can aid elderly patients in ambulating and performing ADL.

The nursing home is an ideal setting for teaching diagnostic and therapeutic approaches to communication disorders in the elderly. The differential diagnosis of communication problems due to aphasia, dysarthria, and/or auditory and visual deficits should be stressed. The nursing home also provides a useful place to refine mental status evaluation techniques. The student's ability to differentiate an elderly patient with normal mental status from one with delirium, dementia, and/or depression is a necessary skill.[18]

The nursing home also allows the medical student to see and participate in the complex decision-making process that occurs in caring for the elderly.[19] Medical, surgical, and rehabilitative decisions concerning the care of the nursing home patient are often complicated by the altered mental status of the patient, by misconceptions on the part of the family and staff about the possible outcomes of medical or surgical interventions, and by attitude of the family, physician, or other health professional toward the prolongation of life when only a few months or years remain. The pros and cons of treating a febrile illness in an elderly demented patient; placing a nasogastric tube in a demented patient who refuses to eat; transferring an elderly nursing home patient to the acute hospital for further treatment when the outcome is not clear; extracting a unilateral cataract and inserting an intraocular lens; and prescribing a lower limb prosthesis, are difficult yet frequently made decisions.

The medical student has the opportunity to assess whether the patient has been appropriately placed in the nursing home.[20] Some of the questions that the student must deal with are the following: 1) Does the patient belong in a nursing home or can he live in his own home? 2) Does the amount of care required necessitate placement at a particular level of nursing home care? 3) Are there reversible components to either the patient's illness or disabilities which will improve his function within the nursing home or allow him to return to the community, supported by family and/or a home care program? 4) What are the risks for the patient and his family of remaining in the nursing home or of returning home?

The student may be confronted with transfer information that is either inadequate or inaccurate.[21] Consequently, he may be forced to piece together a lengthy, complex, and often poorly documented history so that a proper assessment and treatment plan can be made.[22]

The nursing home offers the student the chance to observe and work with other health care professionals with whom he typically has superficial contact during his acute training. The dentist, podiatrist, speech pathologist, audiologist, social worker, and gerontological or geriatric nurse, who work with the institutionalized elderly, have much to teach medical students about assessment, approaches to problems in their respective specialty areas, and methods of professional interaction.[23] The student may also have the opportunity to work with physician's assistants and/or geriatric nurse practitioners, two health professionals who have an increasing role to play in nursing home care. The student should participate in multidisciplinary team meetings where he can directly observe how the nursing home staff deals with the medical, nursing, and psychosocial problems of the patient and his family and learn the approaches and skills utilized in maximizing the effectiveness of the team.[24] Typical team meeting topics are listed in Table 7–1.

The nursing home also presents an excellent arena for learning about altered pharmacokinetics and pharmacodynamics in the elderly, polypharmacy, and the use of drugs in the prevention of illness in the healthy and the ill elderly. The student will become aware of the increased sensitivity of the aged central nervous and cardiovascular systems to drugs, the slower metabolism and excretion of many drugs, and the increased incidence and types of adverse drug reactions, drug-drug interactions, and drug-disability interactions. The use of psychoactive drugs and their interactions with other drugs are especially relevant to the nursing home setting. The medical student will soon realize that there is a significant difference between the 40-year-old, 80-kilogram man taught in medical school and the 80-year-old, 40-kilogram woman encountered in a nursing home, when it comes to drug therapy. The role of immunization in the elderly and, specifically, in nursing home residents, should be emphasized.

Finally, there is no autopsy as humbling to the clinician or the

TABLE 7–1
Typical Team Meeting Topics in the Nursing Home

- Initial evaluation and prognosis.
- Plans for maintenance and/or rehabilitative therapies.
- Unrealistic expectations of family, patient, and/or staff.
- Competence of the patient to make decisions.
- Decisions to resuscitate, withhold therapy, or prolong life.
- Progress in therapy from the viewpoint of all team members.
- Dealing with new problems such as death of the patient (or roommate or spouse), falls, complicated medical or nursing problems, lack of progress in rehabilitation, nocturnal agitation, wandering, and need for restraints.
- Resistance by patient, family or staff to treatment goals.
- Planning for discharge into the community (family and/or community support) or transfer to another level of care (acute hospital, intermediate care, or home care).
- Professional and emotional support of team members in stressful roles.

medical student as one done on a patient for whom he has been caring in the nursing home. Atypical or asymptomatic presentations lead to unexpected pathological findings such as occult neoplasms, ruptured aneurysms, pulmonary emboli, idiopathic hypertrophic subaortic stenosis, or bacterial endocarditis. In up to 30 percent of deaths, no major cause may be found.[25] Neuropathology conferences offer the student the opportunity to learn how normal aging, SDAT, and cerebrovascular disease affect the brain. Clinical correlation with pathological findings is extremely important if the diagnostic abilities of the student are to improve.

Integrating the Nursing Home into the Medical School Curriculum

Rather than exposing the medical student to the nursing home at only one time during his four years, longitudinal exposure at various times and at different levels of sophistication is appropriate. The following are methods of incorporating nursing home based educational programs into the medical school curriculum.

Introduction to Medicine Courses

The Introduction to Medicine courses (first and second year) should have a component that allows the student to explore his attitudes toward aging, old age, and disability through various sensitizing and experiential sessions. The student should be exposed to healthy elderly at screening clinics in senior citizen centers as well as to chronically ill, aged people. Allowing the student to longitudinally follow an older patient through an acute hospitalization, admission to a nursing home, recovery and return home, or lengthy stay in the nursing home, provides insights into many aspects of long-term care. Visits to homebound patients and patients at various levels of nursing home care should also be made. These visits can be complemented by interviews with several patients who are chronically ill or recovering from an acute episode. Didactic and audiovisual material concerning the health problems of the elderly and the role of the health care system in treating the geriatric population can be presented by case example and problem-solving sessions. Based on the previously cited studies, this mixture of healthy, "near-institutionalized," and institutionalized elderly, will improve the student's attitudes and provide a comprehensive exposure to all phases of health and illness in the elderly.

History and Physical Examination Course

Students can learn history-taking and physical examination through interaction with nursing home patients during the second year. My own experience, as well as that of other clinicians and educators in teaching history and physical examination in nursing homes, has been favorable. Nursing home patients are not selected to demonstrate a "museum of pathology." Rather, the student is taught the approaches and skills needed to interview and examine these complex patients. Multiple sensory deficits may make communication difficult and the interview lengthy. "Chief complaints" are usually multiple. The patients' medical histories are long and extra time must be allowed. Physical findings seen frequently in elderly institutionalized patients should be stressed. These include senile purpura, senile angiomas, cataracts, senile macular degeneration, presbycusis, denture ulcers, systolic murmurs secondary to aortic sclerosis or calcification of the mitral annulus, basilar rales, absent knee and ankle reflexes, extrapyramidal syndromes, hemiparesis, tremor, and major functional impairments including altered mental status, gait disturbances, and urinary and fecal incontinence. Most importantly, the student should learn to assess the patient's overall functional status, including both physical and mental aspects.[26]

Ideally, all students should perform a part of their history and physical examination course in the nursing home. This portion would include four to six consecutive sessions allowing the student time to adjust to the new environment and to perform two to four complete histories and physical examinations. Initially, patients who are mentally clear should be selected. As the student's interviewing ability improves, patients with mild to moderate degrees of dementia and disability should be chosen so that the student can refine her/his mental status testing and assessment skills. The problem-oriented medical record should be taught in the nursing home setting, as it is a useful tool to help the student approach multiple acute, subacute, rehabilitative, and chronic problems.[27]

Clinical Clerkship

It is recommended that during the third or fourth year a selective or mandatory clinical clerkship in geriatric medicine be offered. Such an experience would be partially or totally based at a nursing home. The nursing home would also have home care and ambulatory clinics, thereby offering a complete range of services that would allow the medical student to follow longitudinally his patients as they improve, remain stable, or decompensate. Because these patients are medically and psychiatrically complex, it is preferable for the student to have completed the mandatory third-year medical clerkship and a psychiatric clerkship as well. Alternatively, this major clinical exposure to geriatrics could take place before the required third year medical clerkship, when attitudes toward caring for the elderly may be more positive.

There can be two parts to the four- to six-week clerkship—an informal apprenticeship and a formal educational component. The informal apprenticeship would involve supervised primary care, preferably in a multilevel institution that has an acute hospital within the institution or in close proximity. The student can initially be given two to four cases that reflect the typical nursing home population (e.g., patients who have suffered a cerebrovascular accident, a fractured hip, or who have multiple medical illnesses complicated by SDAT, urinary incontinence and/or falling). Each week he will acquire two new cases that are selected because of either the diagnostic or therapeutic challenges involved.

The geriatrician would make teaching and clinical rounds with the geriatric fellow, internal medical residents on a required geriatric rotation, and with medical students, emphasizing the altered presentation of disease, multiplicity of illness, interacting medical, psychiatric and social problems, assessment and maintenance of function, and reversibility of dysfunctions. The student would participate in interdisciplinary team meetings which emphasize the resources needed to assist the elderly patient who leaves the nursing home and enters the community, or vice versa, and the family and community supports that must be integrated to assist him. The student would also be exposed to special departments, such as rehabilitation, dentistry, podiatry, audiology, and speech pathology. The student will make home care visits with the geriatric fellow and take supervised night call at the nursing home.

The formal didactic focus of the fourth year clerkship should consist of modular problem-solving exercises, case demonstrations, selected readings, and formal lectures. A curriculum has been developed and tested on over 100 medical students over a two-year period in a nursing home setting. Specific modules consisting of learning objectives, a pretest, text, problem-solving case histories, and a posttest have been developed. These 15 modules give the student basic approaches to common problems in the elderly as well as detailed presentations of specific areas, including thyroid disease and hypertension in the elderly. See Table 7–2.

Medical Student Research in the Nursing Home

The nursing home provides an ideal place for the medical student to become involved with research in geriatric medicine.[28] Research areas include: (1) nursing home acquired infections, including prevention and treatment of influenza, pneumonia, asymptomatic bacteriuria and others;[29] (2) the epidemiology, diagnosis, treatment, and prevention of urinary and fecal incontinence, gait disorders, falls, delirium and dementia; (3) health care delivery research including: the testing of interventions that are thought to improve or delay decline of functional status; the effectiveness of various health care professionals such as physician's assistants and geriatric nurse prac-

TABLE 7–2
Core of Didactic Material for Fourth Year Clinical Clerkship in Geriatric Medicine

- Concepts of geriatric medicine.
- Interviewing and history taking in the elderly.
- Mental status examination.
- Medication and the elderly.
- Geropsychiatry.
- Rehabilitation of the elderly.*
- Hearing and the elderly.
- Speech and language disorders in the elderly.
- Thyroid disease in the elderly.
- Hypertension and the elderly.
- Geriatric dentistry.*
- Ophthalmology and the elderly.
- Social and economic aspects of geriatric care in the U.S.
- Nutrition in the elderly.
- Podiatry and the elderly.

*Audiovisual (i.e., videotape and audio-slide cassette) components available.

titioners; and methods to more effectively use the nursing home by
decreasing discharges to hospitals, increasing discharges to the community, and/or developing other levels of care or units within the
nursing home that effectively deal with various types of disability,
for example, stroke, incontinence, dementia, or fall units; methods to
improve the transfer of medical information in the institutionalized
and "near-institutionalized" elderly;[30] (4) communication disorders
including sensory deprivation from cataracts, presbycusis and/or
aphasia; (5) pharmacology, including drug discontinuation studies
and studies of drug-disease, drug-disability, and drug-drug interactions; methods to improve the self-administration of drugs should be
explored; (6) prevention of immobility problems, for example, pressure sores, contractures, and muscle atrophy; (7) testing of medical
and rehabilitation devices and equipment, ambulatory assistive devices, and beds and furniture to determine the safest and most functional designs for this equipment in different nursing home settings;
and (8) noninvasive testing, including echocardiography, compute-
rized axial tomography, gait analysis in patients who have fallen,
and blood pressure changes during various maneuvers such as eat-
ing, sleeping, and positional change in patients with orthostatic
hypotension or syncope.

Teachers of Geriatric Medicine

Faculty development is critical to an educational program based in a
nursing home. Medical students who are interested in learning more
about the care of the elderly will lose their enthusiasm and develop
negative attitudes toward the elderly if the nursing home experience
is supervised by physicians who are not interested, not enthusiastic,
not trained in geriatric medicine, or too busy with clinical, administrative, or research responsibilities. Where fellowship programs in
geriatric medicine exist, there will be the traditional educational
cascade of geriatrician-fellow–resident-student on which to base
teaching efforts. Geriatric fellows are generally highly motivated
and provide a fruitful learning experience for medical students.
Allowing interested medical school faculty to make rounds at the
nursing home—instead of at the acute hospital—as part of their
teaching responsibility, is another method for faculty development.
  One of the problems in educating medical students about geriatrics, regardless of the setting, is the shortage of trained faculty who
can be role models and teachers.[31] Despite the increasing number of

fellowship programs, there will clearly be a temporary and probably long-term deficit of formally trained physicians entering the nursing home as teachers and developers of educational programs. These positions must be made more attractive to physicians interested in academic geriatrics through clinical, teaching, and research opportunities.

It is preferable for the directors and faculty of educational programs in the nursing home to have at least half of their time committed to the nursing home either as medical director or primary care clinician. Physicians who are infrequent visitors to the nursing home may not have adequate knowledge of geriatric medicine or the commitment to the institution's educational programs. Nursing home faculty who teach must have academic appointments at the affiliated medical school within a division of geriatrics or general medicine, the department of medicine, or in the department of geriatrics of family practice. It is recommended that a weekly geriatric lecture series directed at geriatric fellows, students, and internal medical residents, who may be rotating through the nursing home, be held at the nursing home as part of a formal educational program. The academic geriatricians and faculty from the medical school and its affiliated hospital would be lecturers and discussants.

Evaluation of Educational Programs in the Nursing Home

Specific learning and behavioral objectives for the nursing home component of a geriatric medical program must be developed. Attitudes, behaviors, and cognitive information should be assessed before and after the nursing home experience so the educational programs can be evaluated and revised.

Conclusion

If the institutional long-term care phase is the sole focus of a medical education program in geriatric medicine, it is likely that the student will acquire a narrow view of our elderly population. In addition, he will not master the approaches, skills, and knowledge needed to deal with preventive or ambulatory geriatrics. If, however, the nursing home functions as the focal point of a wider spectrum of services required by the institutionalized and "near-institutionalized" elderly, the medical student will encounter a continuum of older patients, including those residing in the community and the institution, and be better prepared to care for all of the elderly patients in his future practice.

Notes

[1]R. W. Besdine, "The Nursing Home—A Base for Training Medical Students in Geriatric Medicine," *Proceedings of the Conference on The Changing Needs of the Nursing Home Care* (Washington, D.C.: American College of Physicians, 1980), pp. 79–85.

Butler, R. N. "The Teaching Nursing Home," *JAMA* 245 (1981): 1435–7.

Kerzner, L. J. "Medical Education Opportunities Offered by Long-Term Care Institutions," in Steel, K. (ed.), *Geriatric Education* (Lexington, Mass: Colamore Press [D. C. Heath and Co.], 1981), pp. 41–4.

Libow, L. S. "Geriatric Medicine and the Nursing Home: A Mechanism for Mutual Excellence," *Gerontologist* 22 (1982): 134–41.

Pawlson, L. G. "Education in the Nursing Home: Practical Considerations," *J. Am. Geria. Soc.* 30 (1982): 600–2.

Sherman, F. T. "A Medical School Curriculum in Gerontology and Geriatric Medicine," *Mt. Sinai J. Med.* 47 (1980): 99–103.

Sherman, F. T. "The Nursing Home—A Base for Training Medical Students in Geriatric Medicine." *Proceedings of the Conference on The Changing Needs of Nursing Home Care* (Washington, D.C.: American College of Physicians, 1980), pp. 66–78.

Wright, I. S. "Education in Geriatric Medicine," *Bull. NY Acad. Med.* 54 (1978): 944–50.

[2]K. Callen, S. R. Ingman, and D. J. Lower, "Physican's Attitudes Toward Geriatric Medical Education," *Geront. & Geriatric Education* 2 (1982): 207–12.

[3]G. A. Warshaw, J. T. Moore, S. W. Friedman, C. T. Currie, D. C. Kennie, W. J. Kane, & P. A. Mears, "Functional Disability in the Hospitalized Elderly," *JAMA* 248 (1982): 847–50.

[4]E. W. Campion, A. Bang, & M. I. May, "Why Acute-Care Hospitals Must Undertake Long-Term Care," *NEJM* 308 (1983): 71–5.

[5]National Institute on Aging, U.S. Department of HEW, *Recent Developments in Clinical and Research Geriatric Medicine: The NIA Role.* Washington, D.C.: U.S. Government Printing Office, 4 (NIA 79–199G, Aug. 1979).

Institute of Medicine, *Aging and Medical Education* (Washington, D.C.: National Academy of Sciences 1978), XII. Final Recommendations of the American Geriatrics Society Conference on Geriatric Education. Reichel (ed.) *J. Am. Geria. Soc.* 25 (1977): 510–2.

Department of National Health and Welfare, Medical Education in Geriatrics, Report of a Working Party Health Manpower Report, No. 1/77, p. 11, (1977) Ottawa, Ontario, Canada.

P. E. Panneton, and E. F. Wesolowski, "Current and Future Needs in Geriatric Education," *Public Health Rep.* 94 (1979): 73–9.

[6]C. P. Percy, *Medicine and Aging: An Assessment of Opportunities and Neglect.* Hearings before the Special Committee on Aging, United States Senate, 94th Congress, New York City, NY (1976), pp. 8–9.

[7]Association of American Medical Colleges, *AAMC Curriculum Directory* 1979–80, Washington, D.C., (1979).

[8]E. F. Coccaro, (ed.), *Clinical Geriatric Training Site Directory: Training Opportunities in Clinical Geriatrics/Research in Aging Graduate and Undergraduate Students of Medicine* (Chantilly, VA: American Medical Student Association, Mar. 1979).

[9]M. Rodstein, "A Model Curriculum for an Elective Course in Geriatrics," *Gerontologist,* Summer 1973, pp. 231–5.

[10]P. Coggan, P. G. Hodgetts, J. Holtzman, N. Ryan, & R. Ham, "A Required Program in Geriatrics for Medical Students," *J. Fam. Pract.* 7 (1978): 735–9.

[11]A. R. Somers, S. W. Warburton, & S. Moolten, "Teaching Geriatric Care: Report on an Experimental Second-Year Elective," *J. Family Practice* 6 (1978): 573–8.

[12]L. Greenberg-Libow, "The Development and Administration of a Geriatric Program for Freshman and Sophomore Medical Students," in J. W. Brookbank, (ed.), *Improving the Quality of Health Care for the Elderly* (Gainesville, Fla.: University of Florida Press, 1978), pp. 18–24.

[13]L. S. Libow, & F. T. Sherman, (eds.), *The Core of Geriatric Medicine: A Guide for Students and Practitioners* (St. Louis, MO: C. V. Mosby, 1981).

[14]T. F. Williams, A. J. Izzo, & R. K. Steel, "Innovations in Teaching About Chronic Illness and Aging in a Chronic Disease Hospital," in D. W. Clark, and T. F. Williams (eds.), *Teaching of Chronic Illness and Aging,* DHEW Pub. No. (NIH) 75–876 (1973), pp. 21–32.

R. P. Shannon, "Medical Education at the Monroe Community Hospital: A Long-Term Care Setting—One Student's Experience," in K. Steel (ed.), *Geriatric Education* (Lexington, Mass.: Colamore Press [D.C. Heath and Co.], 1981), pp. 45–7.

[15]R. A. Kane, & R. L. Kane, *Assessing the Elderly* (Lexington, MA: Lexington Books, 1981).

[16]J. G. Ouslander, R. L. Kane, & I. B. Abrass, "Urinary Incontinence in Elderly Nursing Home Patients," *JAMA* 248 (1982): 1194–8.

[17]T. D. Sabin, A. J. Vitug, & V. H. Mark, "Are Nursing Home Diagnosis and Treatment Inadequate?" *JAMA* 248 (1982): 321–2.

[18]G. W. Small, & L. G. Jarvik, "The Dementia Syndrome," *Lancet* (1982): 1443–6.

[19]M. B. Miller, *The Interdisciplinary Role of the Nursing Home Medical Director* (Wakefield, MA: Contemporary Publishing, 1976).

M. B. Miller, *Current Issues in Clinical Geriatrics* (New York: The Tiresias Press, 1979).

L. S. Libow, "The Interface of Clinical and Ethical Decisions in the Care of the Elderly," *Mt. Sinai J. Med.* 48 (1981): 480–8.

[20]T. F. Williams, J. G. Hill, M. E. Fairbank, et al., "Appropriate Placement of the Chronically Ill and Aged: A Successful Approach by Evaluation," *JAMA* 226 (1973).

[21]M. B. Miller, & D. F. Elliott, "Errors and Omissions in Diagnostic Records on Admission of Patients to a Nursing Home," *J. Am. Geria. Soc.* 24 (1976): 108–16.

[22]T. R. Reiff, "The Essentials of Geriatric Evaluation," *Geriatrics* 35 (1980): 59–68.

[23]R. B. Breitenbucher, & A. L. Schultz, "Extended Care in Nursing Homes: A Program for a County Teaching Medical Center," *Ann. Intern. Med.* 98 (1983): 96–100.

[24]F. T. Sherman, "Clinical Problems in Geriatric Medicine: A Team Approach," *Allied Health and Behavioral Sciences* 2 (1979): 1–18.

[25]R. R. Kohn, "Cause of Death in Very Old People," *JAMA* 247 (1982): 2793–7.

[26]L. J. Kerzner, L. Greb, & K. Steel, "History-Taking Forms and the Care of Geriatric Patients," *J. of Med. Ed.* 57 (1982): 376–9.

[27]H. G. Corbus, & L. L. Swanson, *Adopting the Problem-Oriented Medical Record in Nursing Homes* (Wakefield, MA: Contemporary Publishing, 1978).

[28]M. Rodstein, "Contributions of the Long-Term Care Facility to the Medical Care of the Aged," *J. Am. Geria. Soc.* 27 (1979): 410–4.

Rodstein, M. "Research in Clinical Medicine in the Aged (Workshop 1, Part a)," *Mt. Sinai J. Med.* 48 (1981): 557–63.

Rodstein, M. "Research in Geriatric Medicine at the Jewish Home and Hospital for Aged, New York—1944–80," *Mt. Sinai J. Med.* 47 (1980): 96–8.

[29]D. W. Bentley, "Immunization for the Elderly," in R. A. Fox (ed.), *Medicine and Old Age: Immunology and Infection* (New York: Churchill Livingstone, in press.)

[30]F. T. Sherman, & L. S. Libow, "A Portable Medical Record for the Elderly," *JAMA* 242 (1979): 57–9.

[31]L. S. Libow, *Testimony at Joint Hearing Before the Subcommittee on Health and Long-Term Care and the Subcommittee on Human Services of the Select Committee on Aging, House of Representatives, May 17, 1978,* Washington, D.C.: Government Printing Office (No. 95–151); 1978.

R. Kane, D. Solomon, J. Beck, F. Keelor, & R. Kane. "The Future Need for Geriatric Manpower in the United States," *N. Engl. J. Med.* 302 (1980): 1327–32.

8

Functional Abilities Assessment

CAROL L. PANICUCCI*

During the past decade there has been a plethora of articles extolling the use of functional assessments by various health and social care providers for the purpose of determining the needs of older adults, particularly the needs of the frail elderly.[1] Before this era, functional assessments were usually accomplished as part of a rehabilitation plan by physical therapists, occupational therapists, and rehabilitation nurse clinical specialists, and/or nurses developing discharge planning and defining home care goals.[2] Functional assessment meant an evaluation of the individual's ability to carry out those activities generally associated with living independently.

This essay will examine a specific conceptual base of the use of functional assessments and consider the consequences of using a functional assessment tool without simultaneously accepting the total therapeutic model. Instead, the model will be supported as a framework that can assist in meeting the needs of clients, families, and health care professionals for the delivery of adequate health care to older adults.

Clients, family, health providers, and the general community are concerned that individuals can learn, be good parents, be financially able to support their families, and maintain a certain degree of independence. Several assumptions underlie the use of functional assessments for planning a patient's care. First, the ability to perform the activities of daily living and be functionally independent is relevant for all clients. Second, functional ability is a common denominator upon which most persons, particularly the elderly, measure their health status despite disease or disability. Third, the

*The author's appreciation is warmly expressed to Emily Campbell, Kay Engelhardt, and Pamela Lester for their thoughtful reading of and recommendations for various drafts of this paper.

vocabulary used in functional assessment is common and under-standable to both professional and client alike and, therefore, facili-tates communication, especially in defining mutually acceptable goals and therapeutic plans. And fourth, the client's ability to make decisions and to perform in his/her own behalf is as critical, if not more so, than those of the professional if one hopes successfully to implement a specific therapeutic plan.

While actual functional skills have a common meaning in our society, the terms *functional abilities* and *functional assessment* are subject to different interpretations. For the purposes of this discus-sion, the interpretation most generally employed in rehabilitation, nursing, and primary care will be used. To reiterate, functional assessment focuses on evaluating the client's level of ability to per-form those activities associated with independent functioning in the community, which includes the client's role as a contributing mem-ber of society.

Minimally, the health care provider is concerned that clients are able to care for themselves while recognizing they will do so with varying degrees of support. For the aged, self-care is emphasized since the majority are neither employed nor responsible for depen-dent children. A conceptual framework consists of three general levels: (1) control over bodily activities; (2) control over home en-vironment; and (3) control over the ability to function independently in an interdependent world.

Activities one would assess under *control over bodily activities* are the various levels of activity related to mobility, toileting, person-al grooming, and feeding one's self. They are the very basic activities that are crucial for maintaing one's self outside an institution.

Control over home environment on a daily basis involves the activity necessary to prepare meals, keep personal space neat, pro-vide mail and newspapers, entertain oneself, and be capable of communicating with the outside world for social and safety needs. These abilities are the minimal attributes required to maintain a separate household even though an outside support system may be necessary.

Control over the ability to function independently in an inter-dependent world requires that one be able to (1) keep one's finances in order; (2) have the ability and stamina to shop for food and other necessary goods; (3) keep one's home clean, which includes doing or contracting for the performance of heavy chores and household re-pairs; (4) arrange one's own transportation, either by driving, taking public transportation, using community service transportation, or arranging to travel with family, friends, or neighbors.

In addition to these three levels of adult activity, the health care provider should assess two additional areas: (1) The older adult's ability to do those unique activities that the individual considers necessary to be fit and useful, that is, having a yearly garden, canning, taking an annual vacation alone, maintaining a job, or doing volunteer work; (2) the older adult's ability and interest in maintaining a social life, which involves the individual's lifelong level of social functioning. One would not expect, therefore, a minimally socially active young person suddenly to become socially engaged in his/her old age. However, the older adult's self concept can be adversely effected if he or she becomes unable to maintain the customary level of social activities.[3] Maintenance of social life can be divided into two areas. The first is concerned with maintaining social contacts to meet one's own needs by participating in social activities organized by church, clubs, nutrition programs, and recreational groups. The second area is the provision of service to members of one's family or community, either as a volunteer or for a salary.

Cognitive functioning is implicit in these tasks of daily living, and therefore has not been considered as an additional category of functioning. Cognitive processes tend to be categorized in medical language that diminishes the usefulness of functional assessment as a mode of communication between all members of the health care team.

The use of functional abilities as a pivotal concept shifts the health care orientation from one that describes pathology to one that considers the client's abilities to function. It proceeds from the client's strengths, thereby allowing the client, family, and other members of the health care team to cope with the client's health problems without losing sight of his/her need to participate in society as independently as possible for as long as possible. In addition, the processes of collecting baseline data, developing a therapeutic plan, and evaluating the effectiveness of the plan have powerful implications for the type of health care that the client will receive.

When using a functional abilities framework for a client's assessment, one is more likely to use concrete terminology familiar to both lay people and the variously trained health care providers. Client, family, and providers can then effectively discuss baseline data related to the client's present level of functioning and then determine the future functional levels they wish the client to attain.

For example, the providers will need to determine the client's present physiological state and prognosis and evaluate how it will affect the client's ability to attain the desired level of functioning. The provider may offer more objective data, whereas the client and family may furnish qualitatively better information pertinent to usual coping mechanisms, stamina, courage, and will. The acquisition of data related to client motivation and family (informal and formal), community and financial supports is the responsibility of the total team, with each member providing information from his/her own fund of knowledge and expertise. Using a common language to share these baseline data will assist the team in discussing feasible goals and treatment modalities. Incongruities between the goals and treatment plans of different team members, client, family, or various care providers tend to become obvious and more easily open to discussion using such common language. Also, myths associated with the processes of aging will be more easily identified and openly discussed.

Given this orientation to the notion of functional ability, and the use of functional assessment of the older adult in health care delivery, a question arises: Why use functional rather than the typical problem-oriented assessment of the older adult client?

The term "problem-oriented" is inhibiting since it focuses on the client's pathology to the exclusion of his/her abilities and powers to cope. It does not consider the strengths of the client, family, or community. The client, and in unique settings even the family, are objects to be *dissected* by health care providers who tend to recommend the optimal *textbook* therapeutic plan to "patch up" the pathological aspects of the organism. Not only does the problem-oriented method offer the health care providers an unfair advantage in decision making—if not a God-like feeling of control—but this approach can easily lead the provider to focus on each problem in isolation, without ever tending to appreciate the interplay of several problems or symptoms, the client's response to therapeutic regimes, or the impact of the therapeutic regime or other quality-of-life factors. This singleness of focus creates difficulties, not only during the process of making accurate diagnoses and prognoses, but also during the development of individual therapeutic plans that attempt to encompass the total client and capitalize on the client's strengths, motivations, and personal goals. In short, this is not an adequate method for conceptualizing a holistic health care system for older adults possessing unique strengths and abilities while suffering multisystem problems and diminishing stress reserve.

In contrast, the functional ability assessment model considers the areas of client strengths, as well as the client's pathology and other limitations. It provides a normative framework while offering an equal power base to all members of the health care team rather than more power to those members competent in the use of medical categories. The client's functional abilities are evaluated from the perspective of what is normal adult behavior and ability. Any modifications necessary for the client to perform the activities can then be discussed in a reasonably objective manner. In addition, this approach clarifies those activities wherein the client needs assistance, thereby helping providers and family to support, even temporarily, only those activities the client cannot perform. For example, if an elderly person cannot shop at the grocery store this does not mean he/she is not capable of planning meals or preparing them. The service needed, therefore, is shopping. Meals-on-Wheels or institutionalization would be inappropriate ways of meeting this client's needs. The provider can adhere to the old adage, "Do no harm," by not creating unnecessary and possibly permanent dependency.

A description of functional ability assessment would be incomplete without some discussion of the possible dangers that may occur in adopting this approach. Difficulty may arise if team members gloss over or ignore some of the client's problems because of their "poorness of fit" within the therapeutic goals of the group. For example, improved mobility to the point of walking two blocks may be an appropriate goal under most circumstances, but not if it ignores the implications that this activity has for the client's compromised cardiac status.

Another problem may arise with disagreement between various members of the team, that is, client-provider, client-family, and/or family provider. The functional assessment approach leaves open to question who is to set the therapeutic goals. The answer is mutual planning. What if, however, the client's concept of quality of life, and thus therapeutic goals, differ from those of the health care provider, family, or society? For example, an 85-year-old person prefers physical inactivity to protect a failing heart so a manuscript can be finished, while other team members believe the client's quality of life will be better with physical and social activity. Rather than handing down decisions, health care providers must instead use rational and persuasive techniques to help other members of the team arrive at significant decisions. Actually this apparent defect may actually be a strength since the client, if unconvinced of the therapeutic plan's merits, may never implement it. The health care providers and family become more attuned to what the individual believes is necessary for an acceptable life style rather than imposing their or society's values on the client.

The team may agree on a set of goals and methods for reaching them only to discover that they are unable to provide the therapeutic milieu necessary to implement the plan. Critical services may not be available, or the client may lack the financial resources to use them. A feeling of failure may result when goals are not met. A feeling of failure may occur when emphasis is placed upon long-term goals rather than upon a series of short-term goals which culminate in meeting the desired functional level. In other cases, the client may be unable to reach the goals because they are, in fact, unrealistic, the services from family or community are not available, or the client's overall health status changes. It is difficult to accept the need to strive for lesser goals; team spirit and cooperation may consequently lessen temporarily or even permanently.

These pitfalls are rather minor, and ones which the experienced health care provider can often prevent, or at least minimize. The most dangerous pitfall derives from the distortion of the functional assessment from a *model* into a *tool*. This distortion is characterized by the use of functional assessment inventory on a one-time-only basis for the purpose of supporting major decisions such as client placement. This makes functional assessment a tool of the professional, who feels he or she has no need to communicate with client and/or family or other health team members for the purpose of obtaining a complete data base. This misuse of the model is consistent with the American love of standardized scores and pseudo-objective evaluation. The use of such functional assessment instruments in isolation does a disservice to the client, family, health care system, and community.

The one-time-only functional assessment is deficit-based, and provides no suggestion that improvement might be feasible. It implicitly adheres to belief in the irreversible decrement model of aging. This model reflects the belief that aging is a progressive decline in functioning ability that cannot be stopped, modified, or reversed. In contrast, adaptation is a basic premise of the functional ability approach to the care plan of the older adult. This approach maintains that decline with age may be intrinsic or environmental in origin and that, in either case, planned interventions are possible to assist the older adult overcome or modify these changes in order to remain functionally independent.[4]

In summary, functional ability assessment can be a useful approach because it involves the client, family, and all relevant health care providers in the health care planning, management, and evaluation of a client's disabilities. The use of functional assessment and planning based on functional abilities allows clients to be viewed holistically and gives adequate considerations to all strengths and limitations in the client's internal and external environments.

Notes

[1]Balinsky, W., & R. Berger, "A Review of the Research on General Health Status Indexes," *Medical Care* 13 (1975):283–293.

Bloom, M., & M. Blenkner, "Assessing Functioning of Older Persons Living in the Community," *Gerontologist* 10 (1970):31–37.

Fortinsky, R. H., Granger, C. V., & G. B. Seltzer, "The Use of Functional Assessment in Understanding Home Care Needs," *Medical Care* 19 (1981):489–497.

German, P. S. "Measuring Functional Disability in the Older Population," *American Journal of Public Health* 71 (1981):1197–1199.

Gurel, L., Linn, M. W., & B. S. Linn, "Physical and Mental Impairment of Function Evaluation in the Aged," *Journal of Gerontology* 27 (1972):88–95.

Lawton, M. P. "The Functional Assessment of Elderly People," *Journal of the American Geriatrics Society* 19 (1971):465–481.

Leering, C. "A Structural Model of Functional Capacity in the Aged," *Journal of the American Geriatrics Society* 27 (1979):314–316.

McCain, R. F. "Nursing by Assessment–Not Intuition," *American Journal of Nursing* 65 (1965):82–84.

Moore, J. T. "Functional Disability of Geriatric Patients in a Family Medicine Program: Implications for Patient Care, Education, and Research," *Journal of Family Practice* 7 (1978):1159–1166.

Stewart, A. L., Ware, J. E., & R. H. Brook, "Advances in the Measurement of Functional Status," *Medical Care* 19 (1981): 473–488.

[2]S. Katz, A. B. Ford, R. W. Moskowitz, B. A. Jackson, & Jaffe, M. W., "Studies of Illness in the Aged," *Journal of the American Medical Association* 188 (1963):1914–919.

[3]E. Mutran, & Burke, P. J. "Feeling 'Useless' ", *Research on Aging* 1 (1979):187–212.

[4]C. L. Panicucci, "The Older Adult," in D. A. Jones, C. F. Denbar, and M. M. Jirovec (eds.), *Medical-surgical Nursing* (New York: McGraw-Hill, 1978).

9

Hospital Geriatric Practice: New Approaches to Education

STANLEY R. INGMAN AND BERNICE HALBUR

The hospital remains the major setting for the teaching of medical students and residents, regardless of all the discussion about the need to train physicians in outpatient settings. In fact, students and residents feel strongly that the place where major skills and knowledge are to be gained is in hospital rotations. In this chapter, it is argued that training, regarding older persons, must not remain focused on the nursing home or the outpatient experience.

Second, this chapter will argue that a geriatric approach is needed to temper the "typical" hospital care of frail, vulnerable older patients. Third, we hope to show that it is important for medical students and residents to have the opportunity to observe clinicians in hospital settings, who understand and practice a type of medicine that is informed by geriatrics.

The role of the "acute care" hospital in geriatric practice has been examined by a geriatric psychiatrist, Carl Eisdorfer.[1] He cites three reasons why physicians should be concerned about the role of the hospital in geriatric care:

1. Most hospital resources are "oriented toward the sophisticated detection of disease" usually relevant to only a limited number of persons with select diseases.
2. The hospital is currently the most costly of geriatric health care delivery systems.
3. Hospital costs are rapidly increasing.

Eisdorfer goes on to argue for a balance of effort and expenditure between acute care strategies and strategies that employ the full range of services relevant to long-term care, while appreciating that clinical care patterns and norms of practice are difficult to alter. In fact, one barrier to such reform is that physician reimbursement and training are heavily linked to the use of expensive technology. For example, careful histories and physical examinations do not generate the high reimbursement rates which accompany the use of high technological medicine.[2] While complete histories and physical examinations informed by a geriatric orientation would be a progressive step, a geriatric approach and system of delivery must be defined and organized in such a way that health care professionals develop positive attitudes toward older patients and acquire sound patient care strategies. In turn, such professionals should then come to see how such an approach can benefit their older patients and increase patient satisfaction. Thus, the primary focus of this chapter is to offer some guiding principles by which such a geriatric approach could be defined and organized. Before offering those principles, the magnitude and nature of the problem encountered in the hospital will be described.

Magnitude and Nature of the Problem

National health statistics have consistently shown that hospital utilization rates increase with age. Older persons have high admission and discharge rates. In 1967, older persons (65+) represented 24.4 percent of all admissions. Most striking is the sharp increase in admissions for the aged (65+) between 1967 and 1976—60.6 percent as compared to only 10.2 percent for the under 65 age group.[3]

With a higher average length of stay (10 to 11 days for the aged, compared to six days for those under 65), the aged occupy on any day many more beds than their admission percentage would indicate. While the aged represented some 24 percent of admissions in 1976, they occupied more than 36 percent of the beds. In fact, in a visit to a rural hospital in Missouri, 77 percent of the beds were found to be occupied by older patients. However, there are marked regional differences in admission and occupancy rates, as well as differences in average lengths of stay (e.g., the average on the west coast is eight to nine days, whereas the average for such eastern states as New York and Pennsylvania is almost 14 days).[4]

It is helpful then to focus upon the heavy utilizers. Persons 75 years or older accounted for 498 hospital discharges per 1000 population, whereas the 65 to 75 year olds had 305 discharges per 1000 population. Some research seems to indicate that higher admissions rates and readmission rates serve partially to account for this higher utilization.[5]

The high volume of aged being treated in acute care hospitals does not by itself necessitate any remedial action. However, various experts in geriatrics have documented, using a traditional clinical approach, certain iatrogenic problems acquired by the aged as they pass through hospitals.[6] Frequently cited iatrogenic problems in geriatric practice include hospital accidents, hospital-acquired infections, and medication errors.[7] Likewise, Abramson has argued that "the hospital stay ... may actually do harm by unwittingly reducing the individual's capability for social integration.[8] Additional concerns include current negative attitudes toward the aged and their influence on actual treatment; lack of continuity of care, both before and after hospitalization; and the narrow focus of hospital treatment on organ-system disease.

The magnitude and nature of this problem has resulted in pressures to reform the acute care orientation of United States' hospitals and medical centers. In fact, these pressures already have led to several types of organizational reform. For example, one such reform has been the hospice, its goal being to allow people to live out their final days in peace and harmony in a separate inpatient facility, or at home. A second reform has taken place in the stroke units in hospitals. Their intent has been to provide comprehensive rehabilitation to such patients. A third organizational reform has been the public, hospital-based geriatric community care system. In such a system, the hospital takes the lead in the formation of a geriatric approach.

Geriatric Approach to Hospital Care

Despite the suggested role of the hospital in community health care systems, little has been done to clarify a geriatric approach to hospital care and its benefits. In the following section, major principles for such an approach are outlined according to the three typical phases of hospital care. Those phases include the preadmission phase, inpatient care, and the discharge process.

The Preadmission Phase

What constitutes "valid admission" varies from community to community and from physician to physician. Currie and others found that large numbers of patients who were admitted to acute care hospitals were there primarily for other than medical or nursing reasons.[9] They estimated that one-third of these admissions could have been treated at home. Similarly, a study of a Triage project revealed that hospital admissions were significantly reduced by emphasizing home assessment.[10] With enough rural hospitals in Missouri and other states reporting occupancies of less than 50 percent, it is unrealistic to expect hospitals to screen admissions, since this may lower their rate of occupancy. Nevertheless, screening during the preadmission phase in order to prevent nonacute hospitalizations must be seriously considered. Therefore, preadmission assessment should consider the following:

Preassessment to Include Complete Profile. A complete profile of the patient, based on a thorough socioclinical assessment should be conducted with and accompany the geriatric patient. This should shift the emphasis from an acute patient profile to an assessment of the multiple disorders and social-psychological status of older patients.

Record to Accompany the Patient Upon Admission. The physician who makes the decision to admit the patient should, in collaboration with the preadmission nurse/nurse practitioner, develop a problem-oriented medical record which would provide a sound base from which to begin inpatient care. That record should accompany the older patient through his/her hospital stay. Not only should this increase the possibility of continuity of care, it should standardize communication among the members of the health care team in charge of the patient.

Tentative Care Plan to be Developed Prior to Admission. Prior to admission, a tentative care plan for the patient should be developed. This should be based upon the initial multiple disorder and social-psychological assessment. Although this care plan would have to be evaluated during the hospital stay, it should guide the health care team in its treatment decisions. With a tentative care plan, more realistic treatment strategies can be formulated. In fact, the importance of such tentative care plans is likely to increase, as more and more admissions occur via specialized referrals and are turned over to residents/attending physicians who were not the initial primary care physicians.

Inpatient Care

Two general approaches to geriatric inpatient care currently are considered/used in various hospitals. One approach is the geriatric consultation service. This service consists of an interdisciplinary team that accepts referrals from others throughout the hospital. According to Steel, hospitals that have adopted this approach report, on the average, three referrals per week.[11] The advantages of such a consultative service in the hospital setting are multiple: it quickly attains visibility in the midst of a teaching/training environment; it reaches many physicians and patients, thereby maximizing exposure for geriatrics; and it requires only a few initial expenses and generates few costly political struggles over the control of numbers of hospital beds.[12] The major disadvantage of a geriatric consultation service is the tendency for it to become a placement service.[13]

A second approach to geriatric inpatient care is the formation of a separate geriatric health care unit. To date, the core members of such units have been representatives from nursing, general or geriatric medicine, and social work. The advantages associated with a separate geriatric health care unit include the ability to create a special physical/social environment, the ability to develop a therapeutic team, and the ability to create a site for training new physicians. The primary disadvantages include isolation from other health care providers and temporary segregation of older patients from younger ones. Some argue that such segregation may mean "second-class" care. The geriatric health care unit approach is based upon the following guiding principles:

Develop a Geriatric Health Care Team. Not only should core members from nursing, general or geriatric medicine, and social work be part of a geriatric health care team, it should integrate, when relevant, representatives from pharmacy, physical therapy, rehabilitation, nutrition, dentistry, and podiatry. Likewise, the geriatric team should work closely with the admitting physician (and other appropriate hospital personnel). The importance of such close working relations is evident in hospital geriatric units throughout Great

Britain. These relations determine the success or failure in meeting long-term care treatment goals.

Of special importance to the success of such a geriatric health care team is the special geriatric skills of nurses. By attending to mouth care, orientation therapy, and more generally long-term care, nurses will be of special benefit to older patients.

The role of social work in a hospital is often limited to the discharge process, as illustrated in the Beckman and Rehr study of 5,312 older hospitalized patients.[14] That study found most aged who needed the services of social workers were referred late in their hospital stay. However, it is important to integrate early social work representatives into the overall care of older patients. Other types of health care professionals are central to the success of a geriatric health care team; their importance has already been documented elsewhere.[15]

While various members of the geriatric health care team are an important resource for the care of older patients, this team should not take over the care of all older persons. Rather, such a team should assist community physicians with the inpatient care of serious, unstable, vulnerable older patients.

Integrate Some Existing Practices From Physical Medicine and Rehabilitation. Although these areas traditionally have centered on disease/disability, they also have been considered compatible with a geriatric approach. This compatibility is evident in their general concern for rehabilitation and their specific attention to strokes, hip fractures, and arthritis. In fact, these are problems many older patients experience. Thus, attention should be paid to the subtle differences between a disability-oriented and more easily understood rehabilitation unit and a less well understood age-based geriatric unit in the same hospital setting.[16]

Modify Environment to Create a Supportive Milieu. The hospital environment should be adapted to the special objectives and social-psychological needs of older patients. Research has shown that the environment of the hospital has a profound effect on the behavior and attitudes of and treatment toward patients. In the same fashion that pediatric hospital units try to create a conducive environment for the experience of the child, attention should be paid to "humanizing" the hospital environment for the aged. The general emphasis should be on making the hospital a more homelike and less disorienting place for such patients.

With many aged patients spending long periods of time in hospitals, attention also should be paid to environmental issues similar to those in long-term care settings.[17] Many of those issues surround the losses typically experienced by older persons. For example, reduced vision necessitates more light; bright, contrasting colors; and nonglare surfaces. Hearing losses also require attention, because background noises or competing sounds can impede communication with older patients. Taste losses, and the use of dentures by many older patients, should warrant special care in food preparation. Losses of significant and intimate relations highlight the importance of touch in caring for the aged. Nurses should try to enhance the sense of space and time for older patients by fostering "reality orientation" and other similar techniques. In addition, privacy for older patients should be insured during their hospital stays.[18]

The Discharge Process

For many older patients this process goes smoothly; however, even with the recent introduction of more discharge planners and medical social workers to assist in this process, many older patients still receive limited discharge planning and inappropriate post-hospital placement. Thus they often experience hospital readmission. Given this situation, the following guiding principles are offered:

Begin Discharge Planning Early. For realistic discharge planning of older patients, especially the dependent aged, this process should begin at admission. Sufficient time to contact various agents in the community—to know them, to evaluate them, and to match the family or other support system with the perceived and objective needs of the older person—is necessary if the discharge process is to work effectively. In fact, medical and social support should be determined and coordinated in such a way as to enable the patient to remain in or to return as quickly as possible to the community. Such discharge planning may reduce the necessity for long hospital stays and/or readmission.

Preparation of Outpatient Care Plan. A post-hospital care plan for the aged should be developed. Not only should this plan list the detailed steps to be taken after discharge, but a follow-up plan should also be prepared to determine whether the plan was executed and to evaluate its success. Again, this should help to prevent unnecessary, costly readmissions to the hospital.

Preparation of Patient Profile to Accompany Patient. Just as the patient profile should accompany the older patient during admission and the hospital stay, the record should go with the aged patient, whether he is moved to a nursing home, is visiting a home health care agency, or attending day care, day hospital, or another facet of the health service system. The underlying rationale for this is that at any time the most current, complete profile of the older patient should be available. Furthermore, the patient profile should be modified as changes occur in the patient and as care plans are altered. In fact, a patient record sheet summary, which lists problems, test results, interventions, and administered drugs, should be developed as soon as the record of the patient becomes voluminous.[19]

Summary

The focus here has been on the role of the hospital in the care of older persons. Not only is the hospital the setting in which medical students/residents acquire major skills and knowledge, it is the place where they will continue to deal with many aged patients. In fact, a large and ever-growing number of aged are being treated, at high costs, in acute care hospitals. While this situation does not necessitate remedial action, iatrogenic disease acquired by the aged as they pass through hospitals does. This is necessitated by the prevailing negative attitudes of many health care professionals toward the aged (and their influence on actual treatment), the lack of continuity of care both before and after hospitalization, and the emphasis in hospital treatment on curing disease.

In response to the magnitude and nature of this problem, pressure has grown to reform the acute care orientation of United States' hospitals and medical centers.[20, 21] While reform has centered on the development of a geriatric approach to hospital care, little has been done to clarify such an approach and its potential benefits. Thus, we have proffered a few guiding principles for such an approach and do so in terms of the three typical phases of hospital care—preadmission, inpatient care, and discharge process.[22]

Not only are these phases a useful heuristic device for laying out these guidelines, Sherman and Flatley already have proposed and tested a compatible method for studying patients as they move through a hospital stay.[23] In fact, this method was found very useful for detecting patients who had complications with respect to the admitting diagnosis, new diagnosis, or iatrogenic illness. Thus, high quality geriatric care in hospitals will depend on both the principles which guide and the method for studying the treatment of the aged as they pass from admission to discharge.

Notes

[1]C. Eisdorfer, "Care of the Aged: The Barriers of Traditions," *Ann. Intern. Med* 94 (1981): 256–259.

[2]Ian Lawson, "Humanistic Geriatric Education: A Context of Antitheses," Chapter 6 in this volume.

[3]"Hospital Indicator: Utilization Data for Senior Citizens," *Hospitals,* 50 (1976): 47–50.

[4]United States Department of Health, Education, and Welfare, Public Health Services: Health United States (1979). DHEW Publication No. (PHS) 80–1232.

5_____.

[6]A. J. Rosin, & R. V. Boyd, "Complication of Illness in Geriatric Patients in Hospital," *J. Chronic Dis.* 19 (1966): 307–313.

[7]Ian M. Smith, "Acute Care Hospital Geriatrics," in I. M. Ian Smith, G. O. Williams, T. H. Waltz (eds.), *Geriatric Patient Care: Acute and Chronic* (New York: Spectrum Publications, 1981).

[8]A. S. Abramson, et al., "A Therapeutic Community in a General Hospital: Adaptation to a Rehabilitation Service," *J. Chronic Dis.* 16 (1963): 179–186.

[9]C. T. Currie, et al., "Medical and Nursing Needs of Elderly Patients Admitted to Acute Medical Beds," *Age and Aging* 8 (1979): 149–151.

[10]Joan Quinn, "Triage: Coordinated Care for the Elderly," *J. Continuing Education in Nursing* 10 (1979): 1–7.

[11]K. Steel, & Antonelle M. Hays, "The Teaching of Geriatrics in an Acute Hospital Setting," in K. Steel (ed.), *Geriatric Education* (Lexington, Mass.: Colamore Press [D. C. Heath and Co.], 1981), pp. 35–40.

12_____.

[13]Edward W. Campion, "Challenges for a Geriatric Consultation Service in the Acute Hospital," in K. Steel (ed.), *Geriatric Education,* (Lexington, Mass.: Colamore Press [D. C. Heath and Co.], 1981), pp. 221–223.

[14]B. Berkman, and H. Rehr, "The Search for Early Indicators of Social Service Need Among Elderly Hospital Patients," *J. Amer. Ger. Soc.* 22 (1974): 416–422.

[15]William Reichel, (ed.), *Clinical Aspects of Aging* (Baltimore: Williams and Wilkins, 1978).

[16]Richard Lusky, "Rehabilitation and the Elderly: Implications for Geriatric Services," Chapter 14 in this volume.

[17]Stroke Advisory Committee, National Institute of Neurological and Communicative Disorders and Stroke: Bethesda, Maryland.

[18]M. Powell Lawton, *Environment and Aging* (Belmont, CA: Brooks/Cole Publishing Co., 1980).

[19]I. R. Lawson, "Professional Standard Review Organization and Care of the Elderly," *JAMA* 229:3 (1974): 311–313.

[20]L. S. Libow, "A Public Hospital-Based Geriatric Community Care System," *The Gerontologist* 14 (1974): 289–290.

[21] Knight Steel, "Geriatrics for Educators and the Educated," in K. Steel (ed.), *Geriatric Education* (Lexington, Mass.: Colamore Press [D. C. Heath and Co.], 1981), pp. 3–12.

[22] Duncan Robertson, "The Use of an Acute Geriatric Assessment Unit for Undergraduate Education in Geriatric Medicine—The Experience at the University of Saskatchewan," in K. Steel (ed.), *Geriatric Education* (Lexington, Mass.: Colamore Press [D. C. Heath and Co.], 1981), p. 217.

[23] Herbert Sherman, & Margaret Flatley, "Dissecting the Hospital Stay: A Method for Studying Patients Staying in Hospitals," *Medical Care* *XVIII* 7 1980: 715–730.

PART III
THE ROLE OF
THE HUMANITIES
AND CREATIVE WRITING

10

Humanities Teaching and Aging: Issues and Approaches in Medical Education

SALLY A. GADOW

The mandate to all of the disciplines in gerontology is simple. It has been expressed succinctly by Alex Comfort: There is "no pill or regime known . . . [that] could transform the latter years of life as fully as could a change in our *vision* of age and a *militancy* in attaining that change."[1]

Visions, of course, are what the humanities have always been accused of pursuing. Militancy is another matter. But I shall argue that vision and militancy cannot be separated in teaching about aging in a curriculum for professionals who will bear some responsibility for the elderly. Whether virtue can be taught has always been disputed, but there is no question that visions can be taught. Since all students already have some view of aging, Comfort's charge is pertinent: some visions must be *un*learned in order that new ones can be acquired, and for that to occur in a society as heavily socialized against aging as ours, militancy is required. I am not referring (yet) to political activism, but to a more fundamental revolution: an intellectual militancy against dogma in any form (even in humanistic form), and thus a critical exposure of any view—and its derivative practices and policies—that presumes to judge *for* the elderly what the nature and the value of their experience should be.

We find ourselves with a medley of dogmas about aging.[2] At one extreme, which I shall designate the negative end of the spectrum, there still survives the view that aging is a stage of dying, a biological

119

if not also a psychological acquiescence that life is a terminal disease. The negativity of this view derives in part from the general disfavor with which death is viewed. Were death seen as the pinnacle of human experience, aging might acquire a different character.

But even if society availed itself of a positive view of death, another negative vision of aging would be possible and, in fact, is widespread, that is, the view that aging, while not a terminal disease, is nevertheless a disease. This concept of aging as the antithesis of health finds expression in medicine in a deceptively pseudo-objective way, namely, the designation of clinical changes in aging as *deterioration*. To the truly objective observer, however, there is nothing a priori degenerative about the changes in aging unless one uncritically accepts as the only ideal of health the condition that younger individuals manifest. Using that ideal, of course, aging by definition is a profound deviation.[3]

A more charitable view has emerged in which the elderly are elevated from outcasts to underprivileged citizens. When viewed this way—although their age in itself has no intrinsic value for society—they are brought out of the closet to become recipients of our benevolence. But the danger in this view is the danger in the designation of all "handicapped" individuals as special groups needing services: the beneficiary remains subordinate to the benefactor.

An auspicious development is the rise of geriatric medicine, a clinical entity in its own right. From this perspective aging is a unique human phenomenon, worthy of a practitioner's or a researcher's full attention. The aged are not health deviants; on the contrary, they are the "biologically elite."[4] As an elite, they present special strengths as well as special problems that other patients do not manifest. As positive as this development is, it too carries a risk—the possibility that subspecialty medicine would become the model for our basic approach to the aged. This could mean that aging would be of interest as a highly specific class of unusual phenomena, bearing little relation to the more general features of experience shared by persons of all ages. This trend already is evident in attempts to identify sociological and psychological features of aging that distinguish it from the rest of human experience.

Perhaps the most positive of all attitudes so far is the view that the aged are a cultural treasure, a repository of wisdom, an embodiment of history. The growing interest in oral history, for example, regards the elderly as an irreplaceable historical elite. Interestingly, the assumption underlying this regard for the aged is one of modern society's most unquestioned beliefs, that is, the belief that the value of time is proportional to the amount of time. For the elderly, the amount of time already lived far outweighs the time remaining; consequently, the *past* experience of the aged is of greater interest and value to society than the experiences still ahead of them. The positivity of this view cannot be denied; it brings elderly people into the center of efforts to understand our world in terms of its history. But it leaves little room for the 74-year-old woman who insisted, "But doctor, all I have left is my future."

If this spectrum I have outlined depicts the visions presently competing in our regard for the elderly, the situation may be profoundly confusing both for the elderly and for those concerned about them. One redeeming feature of the confusion may be that at last we will be disabused of the dogma that there is an empirically correct way to regard aging, based upon "the facts" and not upon values. As convenient, heuristically, as that bias may be (how could we do research on aging without it?), the moment we acknowledge another level at which aging is a *human*—a personal rather than cellular—phenomenon, we have to concede that a value-free concept of aging is impossible. As Comfort insists, the experience of the elderly is socially, not biologically determined. Visions of aging that remain at the level of biology cannot express the most salient aspects of aging.

Those features that transcend the biological are addressed most directly by the humanities. The particular view of aging to which we subscribe and the militancy with which we solicit new subscribers are basic to our social determination of aging. Dogmatic views of aging are widely advertised and rarely criticized, for example, a commercial in which a youthful-appearing woman challenges the viewer: "Can you guess my age? I am *thirty!*" The humanities are not concerned with entering the market with a new product, a new view of aging to supplant previous dogmas. The purpose of the humanities is to enhance the freedom with which individuals view their experience and the experience of others. To that end, the creation of even a humanistic dogma is defeating, for it limits the ways in which we and the elderly can freely formulate an understanding of aging. Individuals have not, for the most part, been free to create for themselves positive meanings of aging (except for what I choose to call a "false positive" meaning, that is, "you're as young as you feel"). But the remedy for that enforced negativity is not a forced positivity in which we are socialized to unthinkingly applaud aging. The solution, from the humanities' perspective, is a restoration of freedom, in which individuals are allowed to find for themselves the meaning of aging that is the most personally satisfying and consonant with their own beliefs and values. Thus, some may choose to experience aging as a kind of death while others may decide to ignore it altogether. The point is for them to choose their own visions of aging, uncoerced by either negative or positive dogma. In time, we may transcend the poverty of this negative/positive dichotomy that requires that, whatever else we may think of aging, we must be either for or against it. Being "against" it has been the task of the researcher who seeks to slow it, and being "for" it has been the calling of the humanist who often seeks to salvage it. Hopefully we are approaching the point at which we will be free to examine the experience of aging without either presupposition and can thereby arrive at individual understandings of aging that are so rich and complex as to defy reduction to a simple polarity. Thus the role of the humanities is not to provide a new vision, as one might think, misinterpreting Comfort, but to insure a pluralism that prevents any single view from becoming ideology.

My remarks so far have been concerned with the question, why the humanities? Granting that freedom of vision is the *why* of the humanities, now comes the procedural question: *how* is that to be achieved?

There are two levels at which the humanities contribute to a curriculum for health professionals, corresponding to the two levels of involvement with the elderly for which students are prepared: the personal level and the policy level. Students are prepared for work with individual older persons directly, as in geriatric and family medicine, and they are also (ideally) prepared for indirect involvement through program planning, community organization, resource allocation, and so on. Preparation for these two levels—the personal and the political—involves distinct humanities approaches.

The Personal Level

First, we will discuss the personal, or direct care, level which is exemplified in the health practitioner. The objective of humanities teaching in a curriculum, for example, of geriatric medicine is to develop an openness to and an appreciation of the infinite variety of ways in which it is possible to experience meaningfully a condition of human finitude such as aging. How is that appreciation fostered? Three humanities approaches are relevant here.

One is the *historical* study of views and experiences of aging in different eras and cultures.

A second is the *aesthetic* approach, with its focus upon the unique, immeasurable dimensions of experience, that is, the subjective aspects of aging. These dimensions find expression in the art and literature of a culture. But fiction and drama, poetry and biography are not only aesthetic expressions in themselves, expressions that can be distilled for their content relevant to aging. They are also the means of developing in a practitioner an aesthetic regard for aging, as opposed to a clinical or scientific regard.

To illustrate, one aspect of aesthetic regard is an attending to the object, such as a musical composition, with such centeredness in it that a commitment to it evolves. That is, the music is experienced as worthy of regard because of its own, intrinsic value (not its utility). The composition is valued in its wholeness; no part of it is judged insignificant to the integrity of the whole. No phrase in it is too minute to merit attention in order to ascertain its possible meanings. Finally—and perhaps most important in relation to aging—no object, whether sonata, painting, or poem, is so simple that its meaning is self-evident: there are no literal meanings in the object of aesthetic regard because there are no *a priori* meanings.

I have discussed elsewhere some of the possible meanings that the aging body may express as an object of aesthetic regard.[5] In that discussion, I suggest that the "facts" of the aging body can be seen as symbols rather than finalities—symbols of values and meanings that aging may have for the person as a whole. For example, one of the realities of aging is the alteration of smooth surfaces and straight lines, as skin wrinkles and roughens, posture becomes curved, and memory winds around itself. As symbols rather than symptoms these phenomena seem to express

> the finer articulations that are possible in the person for whom reality has become many-layered, folded upon itself, woven and richly textured, a reality no longer ordered in the more familiar linear fashion, but now a world filled with leaps, windings, countless crossings, immeasurably more intricate and perhaps also more true than the world of one-dimensional thought and self-evident distinctions.[6]

A careful application of the aesthetic model in aging would have to address not only the typical processes of aging, but also the much deeper problem of how one is able to develop aesthetic regard for phenomena that elude typification; for the unique way in which individuals shape themselves in aging can hardly be expressed in such general classifications as slowing and wrinkling.

In addition to the historical and the aesthetic approaches, a third humanities approach to the personal meanings of aging is the *philosophical,* specifically, the phenomenological. Here, the phenomena of aging are explored as they are actually experienced *by* the elderly, rather than as they are perceived, valued, and expressed in art and literature *about* the elderly. This poses an interesting problem, however, for many persons who reflect and write about their own experiences do so by distancing themselves from it, surveying their experience with the same objectivity and externally derived expectations with which they address the experience of others. The difficulty of the phenomenological approach reminds us how fragile the phenomena are and how supple the humanities must be to avoid producing an objective characterization of aging rather than presenting the phenomena themselves.

Objectification is a risk in all the humanities approaches I have mentioned. It occurs in part because students are taught via objects: books, films, slides, tapes. The phenomena are packaged for easy consumption. That the life being expressed in those objects still breathes at all when it reaches the classroom is, in most cases, a miracle. For this reason, any humanities teaching about aging must involve the elderly in person. This can be done by including older persons on the teaching staff. It must *not* be done in the usual mode of medical education, using them as "clinical material" to illustrate "conditions" of aging. (The newer model is analogous here, in which health professionals themselves serve as the "patients" in teaching skills such as physical examination.) A phenomenological exploration of aging cannot be achieved without a significant contribution from older persons, both to portray their own perspective and to elucidate the experiences of aging portrayed in literature. Many students have had little, if any, contact with elderly persons and few opportunities to recognize the value of the aged as wise teachers. Thus, a further aim of this approach is to assist in freeing students from inherited assumptions about the disvalue of aging.

Another way to involve older persons is through the performing arts. In our basic humanities course for medical students, for example, we provide the class with a performance by Liz Lerman, director of the Washington Dance Exchange, whose choreography emphasizes roles for elderly dancers. In Lerman's pieces, it has been observed, the senior citizens on stage go through the motions of speaking their lines and dancing, but they are not "representing" mood, character or feeling the way a trained actor or dancer "normally" does. Their real function on Lerman's stage is to be themselves, that is, to present their own reality as a foil against which other ways of being can be measured.

The Political Level

There is another purpose in involving older persons in humanities teaching that relates directly to the second level of professional preparation, the policy or political level. At this level the concern is primarily ethical, as distinct from the other three approaches—the historical, aesthetic, and phenomenological. In keeping with ethical concerns, a teaching staff composed of a majority of elderly persons provides students with an important ethical model in which issues involving the aged are addressed by a group in which the elderly have the principal voice.

Of all the humanities approaches, that of ethics is probably the most familiar to the medical community. The appropriateness of ethics teaching in the preparation of policymakers and politically active practitioners can hardly be challenged, since societal concerns about aging center around not so much ethical issues as ethical outrages—the nursing home industry, forced retirement, economic exploitation, and meager allocation of resources by an affluent society. The objective of humanities teaching at the policy level is therefore more directive than in the preparation for individual health care. There, at the personal level, the goal is an enhanced appreciation of the meanings possible in the individual experience of aging. But when the humanities are preparing professionals for political roles, their aim is more pointed: the identification of ethical principles which, in the form of policy, will assure the elderly the greatest possible freedom as well as assistance in determining for themselves the meaning and value of their experience.

Again, the procedural question: How can that be done in a health curriculum? One way is by involvement of the students in either actual or hypothetical community design, requiring an explicit ethical blueprint articulating the philosophy of the community with respect to the elderly in its midst. The creation of such a blueprint entails at least three ethical principles or commitments. These are commitments to the personal liberties of the elderly, to the individuality of the older person, and to the integrity of the older person's experience. To elaborate briefly:

An ideal community ensures *the personal liberties of the elderly*. This requires that they be involved in all policy determinations affecting them, that they be not only allowed but assisted to be self-determining, both individually and as a group. This means, therefore, that the purpose of advocacy for the elderly is to assist in their self-determination rather than to make individual or policy decisions on their behalf, even though it might be with their well-being in mind.

An ideal community protects *the individuality of older persons* against the forces of stereotyping and standardization. This requires that the elderly, perhaps more than any other persons in the community, have the opportunity for flexible, individually determined work schedules, leisure pastimes, social interactions, and living arrangements. While some older persons may prefer maximum-care situations, others may prefer high-risk situations such as living alone in spite of infirmity or continuing to work in physically or mentally taxing jobs. Some may prefer to associate primarily with older persons, while others prefer to be included in a young and growing family. If human development is essentially the process of defining oneself as a unique individual, then logically, an older person will be even more individual than a younger person and will suffer more from regimens of uniformity, even when those regimens are thought to be in their best interest, as in health care.

An ideal community protects and enhances *the integrity of the older person's experience,* so that the elderly not only are not alienated from the community by reason of their aging, but also are not alienated from themselves through forced dependence and restricted autonomy. This requires a fundamental reconceptualization of aging as a distinct form of wellness rather than a disease or a stage of dying. It also requires that the elderly be offered maximum possibilities for self-care and personal decision making, particularly in regard to health, since health care has a singular potential for estranging individuals from their bodies and selves by delegating most health matters to professionals.

I have emphasized the approach of ethics in the preparation of health care students for political and policy-making roles. Ethics, of course, is crucial also in the personal practitioner-patient encounter, where such issues as truth-telling, paternalism, and euthanasia arise. Certainly students preparing for geriatric practice must address these issues. But I have focused upon ethics in relation to the political more than the clinical level because the political is primary. The ethical problems that a clinician faces will generally be resolved in ways that are consonant with the current philosophy of the profession and society with regard to the elderly. If professional and social policies express commitment to the personal liberties, individuality, and integrity of older persons, it is unlikely that clinicians will be taught to ignore, deceive, or exploit elderly patients. The ethical problems surrounding the elderly are reflected in the clinical setting, but they do not originate there, and cannot be adequately addressed there. The roots of those problems lie beyond medicine, and are finally accessible only through political treatment.

In summary, the humanities approaches of history, aesthetics, phenomenology, and ethics are crucial in cultivating in the practitioner—and thus allowing in the patient—a freedom of vision regarding aging. But for that freedom to be more than illusion, the humanities must also be committed to militancy—that is, the preparation of policy makers who will alter the social realities that presently deny the humanness of aging.

Notes

[1] Alex Comfort, *A Good Age* (New York: Crown Publishers, 1976), pp. 13–18, emphasis added.

[2] Sally Gadow, "Medicine, Ethics, and the Elderly," *The Gerontologist* 20 (Dec. 1980), no. 6, pp. 680–85.

[3] E. Leach, "Society's Expectations of Health," *Journal of Medical Ethics I* (1975):85–89.

[4] J. Jernigan, "The Biologically Elite," Third Annual Medical Aspects of Aging, University of Florida, November 30, 1979.

[5] G. Berg, and S. Gadow, "Toward More Human Meanings of Aging—Ideals and Images from Philosophy and Art," in S. Spicker, K. M. Woodward, and D. D. van Tassel (eds.), *Aging and the Elderly: Humanistic Perspectives in Gerontology* (New York: Humanities Press, 1978), pp. 83–92. Also see S. Gadow, "Body and Self: A Dialectic," *The Journal of Medicine and Philosophy* 5 (September, 1980) no. 3, pp. 172–185.

[6] Berg and Gadow, "Toward More Human Meanings," p. 86.

11

Frailty and the Meanings of Literature

KATHLEEN M. WOODWARD

The United Nations, having designated 1981 as the Year of Disabled Persons, hosted an elegant symposium on literature and the disabled in midfall which was sponsored by The International Center for the Disabled. Engraved invitations were sent to government officials and interested scholars in the humanities. Professors of medical ethics, physicians, and humanists were flown in from around the country to hear distinguished figures in the humanities and medicine—Leslie Fiedler, Herbert Blau, Richard Selzer, and Karl Menninger, among others—discuss the relationships between literature and the disabled. Many in the audience found themselves disquieted rather than comforted by the presentations of the speakers.

Leslie Fiedler spoke about "the *quasi-mythological* role the disabled play in imaginative literature" and reminded his audience—many of whom were primarily concerned with providing services to the disabled and making public policy for the disabled—that "literature *qua* literature is not primarily, or even mainly, intended to inform us."[1] "Much less," he continued, is literature "obliged to show us the error of our ways and move us to right action." Rather, the proper function of literature, he argued, is to alter our ordinary modes of consciousness, releasing in us much that we often repress, revealing the darker aspects of our psyche and the disturbing truths about ourselves. Fiedler insisted that reading literature *qua* literature about the lame or blind will not teach us how to change our attitudes toward the disabled but will—if we are attentive—make us more aware of the deep psychological roots of those attitudes. In a

128

similar vein, Herbert Blau closed his remarks with these rhetorical questions: Doesn't disability do more for literature than literature does for disability? Isn't affliction the deepest subject of literature? Isn't the greatest of our literature about suffering, which is the human condition?[2]

I preface my discussion of frailty and old age as portrayed in Simone de Beauvoir's *A Very Easy Death* and Bernard Berenson's *Sunset and Twilight* with this reference to the United Nations Conference because I see a parallel between what people who are concerned with the disabled expect from literature and what those who are concerned with the elderly expect from it. The conference was organized by well-intentioned men and women who believed that the humanities could help rescue the disabled from contempt, that literature, in particular, could yield positive images of disability, thereby changing our attitudes and moving us to right action. But the speakers at the conference stressed that literature reveals our most profound terrors, our irrational fears of *difference*. Rather than "positive" images of the disabled or of difference, literature *qua* literature offers us, as Herbert Blau put it, "dismembered figures of our crippled or buried selves." Two examples from Western drama—one from an ancient Greek tragedy, the other from a contemporary drama—should suffice: the clubfooted Oedipus of Sophocles' tragedy and the abused, near dead Lucky in Samuel Beckett's *Waiting for Godot*. In these dramas, disability is a sign of a moral crime, as in the case of Oedipus, or an index of the contempt in which those who are different are held by society, as in the case of Lucky.

As for the images of the elderly, it is, I think, the same difference. For the most part, literature *qua* literature offers but cold comfort. Two more examples from the drama will illustrate this point. Perhaps our greatest figure of tragic impoverishment is the failing, elderly King Lear, who in his old age is ruthlessly stripped of status, authority, power, and affection by his two vicious daughters and his untrustworthy subordinates. For Lear, life itself becomes unbearable. As Kent says of Lear, "O, let him pass!" "He hates him/t'at would upon the rack of this tough world/stretch him out longer." Less tragic, more pathetic, are the two aging characters in the ironic *Happy Days,* another of Beckett's plays. Winnie and her silent husband live out their endless hours in meaningless routines in an empty landscape. There is no happy ending. On the contrary, one of the major themes of the play is creeping paralysis. *King Lear* and *Happy Days* convey with great power, on the one hand, and economy, on the other, the suffering and loneliness that old age can bring. More than this, however (to paraphrase Leslie Fiedler), the elderly characters in these two works of great literature play a *quasi-mythological* role. That is, Lear, Winnie and the latter's voiceless companion represent more than the elderly. They symbolize the tragic nature of the human condition, the mutilation of family ties, and the fragmented and crippled nature of Western society. Thus, paradoxically, that is, because these characters represent *more* than the elderly, they tell us *less* about the experience of the elderly than we may wish.

In what follows, I focus on two books in which the elderly characters are not quasi-mythological figures. Both de Beauvoir's *A Very Easy Death* and Berenson's *Sunset and Twilight* present portraits of "real" elderly people who ostensibly stand for nothing over than themselves. De Beauvoir's interpretation of her mother's experience of frailty and terminal illness goes against the grain of her adamant and longheld view of aging as an unrelieved, unmitigated tragic decline. To borrow the title of one of Richard Selzer's excellent books, it is for de Beauvoir a mortal lesson. Through her mother's experience de Beauvoir visits, we might say, a foreign country. Through Bernard Berenson's experience we visit the domain of a frail, elderly person and discover there many surprises.

Mortal Lessons: Simone de Beauvoir and *A Very Easy Death*

De Beauvoir refuses, admirably, to sentimentalize the biological process of aging. The second half of *The Coming of Age* is devoted to the *experience* of aging, what de Beauvoir calls "The Being in the World," or "the discovery and assumption of old age; the body's experience." In old age, she asserts, if one lives long enough, "the body becomes a hindrance" (p. 470), it comes between oneself and the world. It is a barrier. We associate old age with "a dreaded decline," and our "immediate natural desire is to reject it, in so far as it is summed up by the words decrepitude, ugliness, and ill-health."[3] Old age is a stranger. It "inhabits our body," it "worries" us. "Old age reduces strength," she continues, "it deadens emotion."

From this we must not conclude, however, that de Beauvoir does not distinguish between disease and old age. In *The Coming of Age* she calls aging "a new state of biological equilibrium." But it is, admittedly, an equilibrium characterized by powers which have diminished in relation to youth—by failing eyesight, weakened hearing, shortness of breath. It is a precarious, shifting equilibrium which we might call frailty. Recurring throughout *The Coming of Age* are images of vanishing, dwindling, and disintegration. What is fragile or frail is not durable, robust, or longlived. Thus frailty is associated in her mind with shortness of life and nearness to death. As she writes in *The Coming of Age,* "there is truth in the idea of Galen, who placed old age half-way between illness and health." Therefore, although de Beauvoir does not *equate* old age with disease or death, she does insist that there is a powerful connection between the two, a link which many of the most enlightened of us have taken some pains to deny in recent years. It is this equation which horrifies her critics for they wish to dissociate disease and death from advanced old age in order to redeem old age. One way to do this, of course, would be to make sharp distinctions between frailty and disease and then to make a strong argument for the meanings of frailty. It is to de Beauvoir's credit that she refuses to do this.

Thus if the speakers at the United Nations that fall evening in 1981 met resistance because they did not claim great redemptive powers for literature in the service of the disabled—who are indeed often elderly—so Simone de Beauvoir's pessimistic view of aging has outraged many of her readers, including such notable champions of the elderly as Robert Butler and Robert Coles. While her critics often agree with her indictment of Western society's treatment of the elderly as a class, they violently object to her view that aging as a biological phenomenon is necessarily tragic, involving decline and ultimately decay, which our best selves (that is, our active selves) cannot welcome.[4] I might add that de Beauvoir has also been criticized by her most sympathetic of critics—Carol Ascher, among them—for what has been called her lifelong obsession with death.[5]

De Beauvoir's view of old age—which for her is characterized by physical decline and diminished status in the eyes of others—is tragic. She believes that the only noble recourse is to fight against it. As she puts it, "for those who do not choose to go under, being old means fighting against old age" (p. 450). Thus, in a sense, for de Beauvoir old age is the supreme test of one's heroic powers. As she wrote in an early philosophical tract entitled *The Ethics of Ambiguity,* the "tragic ambiguity of the life of man is to recognize our mortality; it is in the knowledge of the genuine conditions of our life that we must draw our strength to live and our reason for acting."[6] The word *"acting"* is central here. As an existentialist, de Beauvoir believes that in old age we will continue to define ourselves only by our actions, that is, our projects, and frailty threatens to turn us inward, away from the world.

It is against de Beauvoir's contempt of frailty and old age that we must read her moving memoir of her mother's death by cancer. Entitled *A Very Easy Death,* this short book—published some six years before the appearance of *The Coming of Age*—is the finest testament to date of de Beauvoir's powers both as an eloquent writer and as an astute observer of character and of everyday life. It also reveals that de Beauvoir, when faced with the complexities of a unique, single life, finds her attitudes toward aging—her theory, that is—inadequate to measure that experience completely.

A Very Easy Death opens with the hospitalization of de Beauvoir's 77-year-old mother for a broken femur (she fell in the bathroom) and the subsequent painful discovery of her advanced terminal cancer. We know from *The Coming of Age* that her mother had suffered for years from arthritis. Thus, the context of her mother's injury (the broken bone) and her terminal disease (her virulent cancer) is frailty. Yet de Beauvoir would never admit that we die of old age. Whether or not it might be in some cases *correct* medically to say that we die of old age, this is not acceptable to her in *human* terms. In the last paragraph of *A Very Easy Death,* de Beauvoir confesses that before her mother's death she had not understood how a 50-year-old woman could be overcome by the death of her mother. Intellectually it seemed quite natural—a woman that age was of an age to die. She opens *A Very Easy Death* writing of her mother's hospitalization: "I was not very much affected. In spite of her frailty my mother was tough. And after all, she was of an age to die."[7] But with the death of her mother de Beauvoir realizes, profoundly, that you do not die from old age: "you die from *something* . . . there is no such thing as a natural death: nothing that happens to man is ever natural, since his presence calls the world into question." This, for her, is the tragic ambiguity of our existence.

The drama of *A Very Easy Death* turns on de Beauvoir's moral dilemma as a daughter who must take responsibility for consenting to a first operation that may prolong her mother's life but will also assuredly prolong her suffering. Should her mother be operated on? In principle, de Beauvoir had long been opposed to what we would call heroic medical measures. But when confronted with the imminent death of her mother, she refused to allow her to die so easily. It was literally unthinkable; she consents to the operation without thinking, without question. Tormented by the consequences of her decision, she nonetheless concludes in retrospect that she could not have decided death for her mother; for those 30 days had brought joy as well as misery. In this respect de Beauvoir's book illustrates perfectly

Jacob Bronowski's view that our best literature does not offer us parables of right action but rather reveals the ambiguities and complexities of our experience.[8]

I will not dwell on the interesting ethical questions raised by this dilemma or on de Beauvoir's blunt indictment of physicians and medical technology, which is a central theme of the book. Rather, what most concerns me is her evaluation of her mother's final days. For de Beauvoir, those days are a revelation of the precious nature of life. She is moved by her mother's responsiveness to the often unnoticed pleasures of everyday life. As de Beauvoir writes:

> What touched our hearts was the way she [her mother] noticed the slightest agreeable sensations: it was as though, at the age of seventy-eight, she were waking afresh to the miracle of living. While the nurse was settling her pillows the metal of a tube touched her thigh—"It's cool! How pleasant!" . . . She asked us to raise the curtain that was covering the window and she looked at the golden leaves of the trees. "How lovely. I shouldn't see that from my flat!" She smiled. And both of us, my sister and I, had the same thought: it was that smile that had dazzled us when we were little children, the radiant smile of a young woman. Where had it been between then and now?[9]

On the last page of *A Very Easy Death*, de Beauvoir confesses that her mother "encouraged one to be optimistic when, crippled with arthritis and dying, she asserted the infinite value of each instant."[10] De Beauvoir comes as close to expressing religious sentiments as she does anywhere in her work when she writes of the final moments of her mother's life: "For myself I understood, to the innermost fibre of my being, that the absolute could be enclosed within the last moments of a dying person."[11] Furthermore, de Beauvoir concludes that it is precisely in the last weeks of her mother's life, when she is at her most frail, that she becomes more herself.

The first and most important question is whether, under personal pressure, de Beauvoir romanticizes frailty and illness. In my opinion, she does not, as Virginia Woolf for example is tempted to do in her essay "On Being Ill." I quote from its opening sentence:

> Considering how common illness is, how tremendous the spiritual change that it brings, how astonishing, when the lights of health go down, the undiscovered countries that are then disclosed, what wastes and deserts of the same a slight attack of influenza brings to view, what precipices and lawns sprinkled with bright flowers a little rise of temperature reveals, what ancient and obdurate oaks are uprooted in us by the act of sickness. . . .[12]

The claims that Fiedler made for literature *qua* literature—it alters our ordinary mode of consciousness—Woolf makes for illness; but, as her style reveals, she sentimentalizes sickness. Woolf's long opening sentence breathlessly enumerates one marvel after another which illness brings—its "undiscovered countries," its "bright flowers." De Beauvoir's style, by contrast, is plain and matter-of-fact. Her descriptions of her mother's illness and disfigurement are exact and painful—neither clinical, nor lyrical.

Although de Beauvoir's temperament is tragic, she would not submit that wisdom necessarily comes from suffering, as Greek drama tells us. However, de Beauvoir's interpretation of the fruits of her mother's illness is curious. Her reading of her mother's final days reveals more about *herself* than about her mother's experience or, indeed, about the relationships between frailty, illness, and insight. In other words, although de Beauvoir did see her mother's final days as positive, as redemptive of her life, we must ask why; for we must always be on guard when people take it upon themselves to speak for others.

What precisely does de Beauvoir mean when she tells us that her mother became more herself during the last month of her life? Why does de Beauvoir admire her mother's behavior during the last 30 days? Here we will do well to remember that *A Very Easy Death* is composed of short chapters which resonate between the near past (the narrative of her mother's illness), the distant past (de Beauvoir's astute appraisal of her mother's life and character), and the present (the analysis of the meaning of the relationship between those other two levels of time). We learn in meditative flashbacks that de Beauvoir's mother had a sensuous nature that not only went unfulfilled after her husband turned to other women but, worse, she grew slovenly and contemptuous of her own body. We also learn that she was a practicing Catholic who complied with the regimen of its rules and lived her life, duty-bound, for others, "corseted in the most rigid of principles." All her life, she writes, her mother "*lived* against herself. She had appetites in plenty: she spent all her strength in repressing them and she underwent this denial in anger."

As we might expect, de Beauvoir is critical of the values by which her mother lived her life. We might not be surprised, therefore, to learn that de Beauvoir regards her mother's frailty and illness as the very conditions which set her free from her lifelong constraints and turned her toward the values de Beauvoir respects. It is the very self which her mother had repressed her entire life which was (figuratively) "deformed and mutilated." It is this self which is liberated because of her (physically) deforming illness. De Beauvoir is pleased that her mother does not ask for the last rites from the church. She regards this as an act of courage. Her mother's illness, she writes, "had quite broken the shell of her prejudices and her pretentions." She becomes more self-assertive, less regarding of others. She discovers "the pleasures of being waited on, looked after, petted." Even more oddly, de Beauvoir interprets her mother's increasing consciousness of her body and her physical nature—which comes with frailty or illness— as liberating her from a long past which denied the body. As she writes: "Maman had not been in the habit of taking notice of herself. Now her body forced itself upon her attention. Ballasted with this weight, she no longer floated in the clouds and she no longer said anything that shocked me." Thus, whereas in *The Coming of Age* de Beauvoir associates the decline of the body as coming between oneself and the world, here it is the body which de Beauvoir believes restores her mother to her true self.

My reading of de Beauvoir's interpretation of her mother's last days suggests not only the limits of theory when confronted with the texture of a unique life but also the limits of interpretation: we inevitably impose our values on the experience of others.

Thus, in closing, I turn to a first-person account, to the detailed autobiographical record in diary form of the last thirteen years of the life of the distinguished art historian Bernard Berenson, who lived the many years of his life before he died at the age of 93 in a comfortable villa in northern Italy.

The Experience of Frailty: Bernard Berenson's Diary

Sunset and Twilight, a book edited from Berenson's voluminous diaries after his death, runs over 500 pages. It is a candid, unflinching record of Berenson's feelings, his thoughts, and his health as it steadily deteriorated.

As Berenson notes, at the age of 82, "How is one to understand without experience, and how is one to procure the experience before body and mind have been matured for it? And real conviction in things human comes from experience and almost never through dialectics."[13] In great part, this experience is of a failing body. "My earthly tabernacle," he writes with humor—a gift de Beauvoir does not share with him—"is too uncomfortable to live in. It leaks, it crumbles, it breaks away, now part of the roof and now a bit of the wall. . . . It is no longer habitable." He complains of physical exhaustion, a failing memory, and weakened concentration. At times, all his effort must go to merely keeping alive: his present career and a fulltime job. As he wrote on November 24, 1951, when he was 87:

> I recall writing not much more than a year ago that every part of me was in tolerable condition. I fear I must write the opposite now. Memory for names gone entirely, and vocabulary in English even diminished. Absent-minded, and restricted horizon, although brain still active but in ever narrowing circles. Aches wherever I touch my body, from skull to toe; shooting pain in my insides. Hernia, threatening hemorrhoids, feeling of repletion, accompanied with slight nausea. Nose dripping or sneezing. Throat, coughing and spitting. Wake after four hours and for better part of an hour sneeze, cough, and spit till I fall back exhausted and doze. Get tired after a half hour's walk or concentrated work.

But there are rewards, he believes, three of which I mention here. First, after 70 years of experience as an art expert, Berenson affirms that he can "see deeper and clearer than ever before, and see beauty where I did not see it before, and enjoy it in actuality and in artifacts as never before."

Secondly, through his own experience of periods when he did not *desire activity,* when he was content merely to be, he comes to have new pleasures and, importantly, to understand and accept this in others. I find one of the most interesting sections of his diary to be his confession of irritation with his late wife for not being active, for being content to doze through the day doing nothing. Several years later he writes: "Day before yesterday I enjoyed complete relaxation, every bit of me, inside and out, at rest. My mind did not work at all, although I was aware of how happy I was, as perhaps never before in memory. I was not thinking. I was not questioning. I was not dozing or dreaming. I was enjoying perfect bliss." A month later he writes, astonishingly so for this intellectual, "I have hated the idea of existing as a vegetable, or less, but it now looks as if I could end by not minding it at all."

And thirdly, through his last years, Berenson relies totally on the care of others who love him. Rather than struggling for independence, he allows a sweet dependence to flourish. This is precisely what the geriatrician Ian Lawson has suggested we must cultivate— what he calls "an ecology of dependence." And for Berenson its blessing is this: "To encounter such love, such devotion, such self-sacrifice, is an experience worth paying for with all I have been through during this crisis." The love of others is the greatest gift of others.

Berenson concludes that "all experience that does not cost others too much is worth having for its own sake, pain if not *ultra vires,* and pleasure even if dulled, dimmed, and muted." He asks rhetorically, "Do we always get aware of things through privation, and remain unaware when we abound in them?" These are the meanings of frailty for him in his old age.

Notes

[1]Leslie Fiedler, "Pity and Fear: Myths and Images of the Disabled in Literature Old and New." Symposium, sponsored by the International Center for the Disabled in collaboration with the United Nations, New York City, October 27, 1981.

[2]Herbert Blau, "The Afflictions of Literature." Symposium sponsored by the International Center for the Disabled in collaboration with the United Nations, New York City, October 27, 1981.

[3]Simone de Beauvoir, *The Coming of Age,* trans. Patrick O'Brian (New York: Warner Paperbacks, 1973), pp. 60, 447 and 596.

[4]Many of those who admire Dylan Thomas for his rage against the dying of the light charge de Beauvoir with *bitterness* toward aging. This patent contradiction, I suspect, has to do with blind stereotypes about gender: women are expected to accept age with grace; men—like the heroic Santiago in Hemingway's *Old Man and the Sea*—are expected to fight against age with vigor.

[5]Carol Ascher, *Simone de Beauvoir: A Life of Freedom* (Boston: Beacon Press, 1981).

[6]Simone de Beauvoir, *The Ethics of Ambiguity,* trans. Bernard Frechtman (New York: Philosophical Library, 1948), p. 9.

[7]Simone de Beauvoir, *A Very Easy Death* (1964), trans. Patrick O'Brian (New York: Warner Paperbacks, 1973), p. 17.

[8]Jacob Bronowski, *The Identity of Man* (Garden City, New York: Natural History Press, 1965).

[9]Simone de Beauvoir, *A Very Easy Death,* p. 60.

[10]———. p. 123.

[11]———. p. 174.

[12]Virginia Woolf, "On Being Ill" (1973), in *The Moment,* (New York: Harcourt, Brace, Jovanovich, 1948), p. 9.

[13]Bernard Berenson, *Sunset and Twilight: From the Diaries of 1947–1958,* Nicky Mariano, ed. (New York: Harcourt, Brace and World, 1963), p. 18.

12

The Aging Experience as Reflected in Creative Writing

RUTH CAMPBELL

> I think upon it in quiet. There is ample cause for joy
> and ample cause for lamenting.
> Po Chui (on the birth of a son in his old age)

For the past three years, about 30 men and women have been meeting weekly in two separate groups at an outpatient geriatric clinic at the University of Michigan in Ann Arbor to read to each other the memoirs, fiction, poetry, and essays they have written at home during the previous week. The writers range in age from mid-sixties to 90, with the average being somewhere in the late seventies. There has been a remarkable amount of stability in group membership with few dropouts, and a sufficient flow of new members for each group to maintain 12 to 18 members. As the director of one of the groups, I find it difficult to begin to describe what they do and how they do it because my role is to listen, to appreciate, to agree or disagree with opinions expressed, and to receive, like a gift, the array of writing offered.

The format does not vary; we begin with the first volunteer to read, and proceed around the table. If someone has not written that week, he or she may say there wasn't enough time or there is a work in progress but as yet unready. Frequently, those who have not written will have a good story to tell, usually stimulated by something one of the group members has said. As we go around the table, and one person reads in the soft accent of southern Missouri, another in German-tinged English, and the next in New Yorkese, we move with the voices from past to present, from politics to philosophy, from great-aunt Susanna to Mosetta the duck who was discovered the other day, like her namesake Moses, hidden in the tall grass outside Mary Grindstaff's house.

For me, part of the pleasure comes from being a legitimate member of the circle. When I was seven or eight, I would sneak downstairs at night to sit on the steps behind the kitchen door. There, unseen, I would huddle, arms wrapped around my knees for warmth, and listen to the roaring voices in the kitchen. We lived with my grandfather, grandmother, and my father's unmarried sister in a three-story house above our grocery store. It was the custom every night about nine, after the store closed, for the family to gather in the kitchen to talk and to eat huge delicatessen sandwiches and soup bowls of ice cream. Overweight and argumentative, they carried on loudly, telling stories about all the relatives and battling with each other. Soaring above the tide of voices was my grandmother's booming Yiddish. Sometimes, forgetting myself, I'd take sides and shout my opinion, whereupon I'd be sent immediately to bed.

Writers as diverse as Margaret Mead, Sharon Curtin, Alex Haley, and Eudora Welty grew up listening to the stories of their elders. From them they learned the secrets and anecdotes of family history and from them they felt a sense of community that lingered in their memories the rest of their lives. Berg and Gadow write that "the humanities are concerned with creating or uncovering new human meanings for our experience—a way of understanding an experience which enhances the value of the experience for the individual and at the same time preserves the element of freedom in human existence by opening a door to new possibilities."[1] The writing groups perform this function in three ways: (1) through writing, most often autobiographically, the writers select from their experience in a more conscious fashion than they would during oral reminiscence and, thus, recreate their own identities; (2) through reading their own words, they take the risk of opening up their lives to the reactions of the group, often discovering new aspects of these experiences and their reactions to them; (3) through listening to others, memories are stirred and forgotten bits of history revealed to themselves.

At the beginning, none of us really knew what would happen. Leon Edel tells us, "Proust, in the footsteps of Bergson, discovered for himself and demonstrated how a calling up of the past establishes man in time, can give him identity and reveal to him the realities of his being."[2] That was a gift we did not expect. The second gift was closely related to what Victor Turner describes as "communitas," a connection of social unity characterized by undifferentiated social status. It is "my writing party" to one, a "family" to another. One member says, "The group membership turned out to be so miscellaneous, such honest genuine people and so sincere, that I never want to give it up. We are very different but perfectly integrated and I love every one of the others."

The members of the writing group do not view themselves as old people. In the group they are writers, concerned with the effort of finding the right words, of juggling reality and imagination. Yet their old age is not insignificant to their work. There is a richness to the material because it spans not only the 70 or 80 years of their own lives but the remembered lives of their parents and grandparents, the wealth of books read, events witnessed, cultural values and ideas inherited. If their writing is any good, it will have a timelessness which will transcend the fact of the writer's age. Therefore, the problem becomes one of delineating the special attributes of writing late in life without putting their writing into a neat little box labeled "memoirs of an old person."

The popularity of groups of this sort has spread widely in recent years. In 1972, when Marc Kaminsky began doing poetry groups for the Jewish Association for Services for the Aged in New York, he felt, at first, as if he were working in the dark; what he was doing could not be characterized as poetry therapy or poetry workshops: "They were quite definitely poetry groups. They were the place where we found the person in the poem and the poem in the person."[3] In his wonderful book, *What's Inside You, it Shines Out of You,*[4] he described the process by which the group wove its memories, dreams, thoughts, and feelings into poetry. Since then others have written of their experiences conducting poetry and writing groups in nursing homes, senior centers, union halls, churches, and universities.[5] A catalogue compiled for the Policy Symposium, *The Arts, the Humanities and Older Americans,*[6] lists programs offered throughout the country where older people come together in groups, both writing and humanities, to share life histories, written and oral. The testimony of people involved in these groups is impressive. One woman wrote that her writing group "raised me from the depths of blackest despair and thoughts of self-destruction to a whole new person again who can face each day and look forward to its arrival. . . ."[7]

The theoretical foundation for many of these groups comes from an interest in reminiscence and aging stimulated by Robert Butler's work on the "life review" process. The perspective gained through a review of the past events of one's life may be a way of achieving what Erikson sees as the task of old age—making sense of what has passed and coming to a kind of acceptance of it, the resolution of the "last" crisis between "integrity" and "despair."[8]

Meyerhoff and Tufte also see reminiscing as a way of integrating one's life experience.[9] Meyerhoff's "Living History" classes were an attempt at "ordering, sorting, explaining—rendering coherent their long life [sic]. . . ."[10] As the elderly Jewish men and women sat around the table telling their stories, sharing their dreams and wishes, they became witnesses to each other's lives. "Listening was not these people's custom," Meyerhoff tells us (Is listening *any* people's custom, one might ask?), but the group provided an audience which gave meaning and significance to the tales the people told. The advantage a structured group has over an informal conversation is that the rules are quite clear: "You listen to me and then I listen to you."

Yet there is some disagreement among researchers on both the frequency with which older people reminisce and the positive value that reminiscence holds for them. LoGerfo points out that some studies recorded only minor differences among age groups in the temporal setting of thoughts or daydreams, while other studies suggested that the frequency of reminiscence does increase markedly with age.[11] There are also differing opinions on the relationship between reminiscence and psychological adjustment. LoGerfo suggest that the inconsistent findings are in some part due to the fact that the researchers used no standard operational definition of reminiscence, and thus measured widely different populations among the elderly with widely different methodologies. LoGerfo identifies three distinct though overlapping forms of reminiscence: (1) informative (Meyerhoff's "Living History" classes for example); (2) evaluative (Butler's "Life Review" concept); and (3) obsessive (occurring when the past is for some reason unacceptable and the person becomes agitated, depressed, or suicidal as he repeats the details of these past events).

According to research done by Revere and Tobin, the "modal" style of reminiscing for the aged is to "mythicize" the past in order to recreate a unique, not necessarily realistic, history for themselves.[12] Ronald Blythe, writing about the aged in an English village, observes that "one of the reasons why old people make so many journeys into the past is to satisfy themselves that it is still there."[13] However, it is clear from Blythe's interviews that he has encouraged these journeys into the past through the questions he has asked. Surely he was interested in comparing the past with the present; he wanted to hear stories of what the village used to be like. A 90-year-old woman I know complained about the student visiting her weekly on assignment from a psychology of aging class. "All she wants to hear about is the past. What I really want to talk about is what is going on in Iran."

Anyone who has ever overheard the conversation of children as they recapture highlights of their past—games almost won, tricks played on parents, heroic exploits of classmates—cannot believe that only old people are involved in their past. They simply *have* more past to begin with. When I conducted a writing group in a federal prison for men aged 19 through 25, the sad fact emerged how little of life they had experienced. Despite flaunting the terrible things they had seen and the unconventional behavior they had displayed, it became obvious after the first burst of glory that they had run out of things to write about—both their imaginations and their experiences had failed them. The older people in these two writing groups, after three years, show no signs of running out of material, nor do they become less interesting. An incident unthought of for years is as likely to reappear as a recounting of what happened yesterday.

Older people often do have more time to devote to the retelling of past events, and there is no denying the special significance of reviewing one's life after many years of living. The important question is what we, as friends, relatives, gerontologists, and humanists are willing or eager to listen to. In an attempt to elevate the image of older people in our society, are we too eager to emphasize their connection with our past rather than to acknowledge their vivid appearance in our present and future? A further complication is that for some older people the present is not interesting and its limits too severe to provide a spur to the imagination.

Writing, as a form of growth, is not confined to older people of course. Arthur Koestler has written that "all creative activity is a kind of do-it-yourself therapy, an attempt to come to terms with traumatizing challenges."[14] The psychologist Ira Progroff devised his Intensive Journal system so that people could have a structured method for looking at their lives. Dreams, fantasies, and wishes are all part of this effort to expand and actively explore awareness of one's own life process. Anais Nin knew that creativity and self-therapy were interrelated, and her remarkable use of the diary provides a model for what Tristine Rainer describes as the "New Diary," a method for exploring thoughts and feelings, recording impressions, and charting one's progress.

Aside from using one's life as material for diaries, fiction, and poetry, writers have published memoirs at all ages, especially if they are celebrities. John Kenneth Galbraith, speaking about his recent autobiography written at the age of 73, remarks that politicians are too hasty to rush into print. Memoirs should not be written, he says, until the person is old, removed from immediate experience, and able to put his own life and the history of his time into some perspective. With this caution about what is unique about the writing of older people and what is shared with those of all ages, I should like to describe the two writing groups at Turner Geriatric Clinic in Ann Arbor and why they write, what themes are conveyed in their writing, and what the outcome is for those who participate.

Development of the Group

I organized the first group because as a social worker I kept hearing— in the midst of an interview—the expression, "I could write a book.... If you only knew what I've gone through." Why didn't they write books? The two great advantages of aging (which can, as well, be two great disadvantages of aging) are the increase in unallocated time and the quantity of "material" each person has collected. Yet writing is a lonely task and most people find it convenient to procrastinate, to wait for the "perfect time." When you are 75 and that time has not arrived, you need, as many of the writers in the group have remarked, "a push." I decided to provide that "push" in a local newspaper for senior citizens:

An article in the newspaper carried the headline, "Do you want to write a book?" and asked interested people to call the clinic. After twelve people had called, the group was formed; that was at the end of March in 1978. Within a few months, it grew to 15 members and a new group was formed to accept the overflow. At the first meeting I stated the following reasons for forming the group: (1) to encourage creativity; (2) to get a better understanding of one's own life; (3) to preserve and pass on memories; (4) to share one's experiences with others and (5) to interpret what has happened and reflect on its meaning as time passes.

The members themselves came with varying goals. Agnes Fries, at 84, wanted to "write down information about my family and my husband's family for the benefit of our children and their children. I myself have often wished, during my later years, that I knew more about my elders. When one is young, one is so busy living actively that it doesn't often occur to ask while some of the elders are alive. My own children seem to me strangely uncurious about their origins. I wanted them to ask, which they seldom did, but the time will come when they will want to know." She has since presented her children each Christmas with photocopies of her writings illustrated with old family photographs. Thus, we see Agnes as a young girl standing beside her father's desk, the history and meaning of which we have just read.

This sense of having lost a part of one's own history was echoed by others in the group. Antonie Hermann came to this country from Germany when she was 18. She spent most of her life working as a housekeeper for a farmer in Michigan. When he retired, they both moved to town where she discovered that others share her love for reading and her urgent need to keep learning as a kind of remedy for her lack of formal education.[15] She writes, "One of the regrets that I carry around with me is that I never asked my mother or any other relative more about their lives, what they remember most vividly and what was the high and low point of their years. For instance, what happened to the four boys my mother bore, who all died before the age of two? My grandfather Norbert was a skilled tradesman, a tinsmith. What happened to his small store and why did it all die?"

These two women, however, disagree on their motivation to write. Mrs. Hermann writes "because I am a stranger to myself. What is it that makes me function? What are my good points, what are my hang-ups? I have a double dose, German and American. Who am I? What am I? What am I today and where am I going? Born of man and woman, I am aware of myself as a link to eternity, and that is what writing does for me. It is a key; it is a key that unlocks the door to truth and muted ecstacy."

Mrs. Fries, on the other hand, says, "As for therapy, I don't think that writing about my family history does anything of that sort for me. I am an inner-directed person and my dour Scot's background won't let me 'tell all.' I don't feel that I need therapy. I am usually busy, usually happy, and I manage to push back into my unconscious the thoughts I don't like to have. I know that some of the present theories suggest that it is harmful to do this, but from my own personal experience I cannot believe that it is true for me."

Lewis Kellum, a retired geologist, kept detailed diaries during his fascinating career, which included searching for oil in the wild lands of Mexico. But his children found them dull and wouldn't read them. With help from the group, the stories he distilled from the diaries are now exciting accounts: in one, money is dropped from an open cockpit biplane into a Mexican jungle, the author's first and most frightening ride in an airplane. He writes of a colleague's exploits forty years ago and of horse thievery in 1981. Even his children are now interested in what he writes.

Some people joined because they wanted to be published. Others had always dreamed of being writers, and yearned to create short stories and poems. Jack Schwartz didn't want to write at all, but his wife forced him to come with her. For many years they had worked together running a bakery; when they retired, she wrote a book about their customers and their struggles to survive through union battles and depression. She came to the group eager to continue writing and with the hope of having her book accepted for publication. She also hoped her husband would start writing; he has. He writes of shopping with his wife, and "wearying" of her indecisions, sinking into a chair where a fantasy seizes him. Balls of yarn rise off their shelves, weaving and spinning a multicolored dance just for him. But Jack's favorite subject is his wife:

> Morty and I were walking on Madison near 86th Street on a hot July day—to be exact the first day of the month. It was a typical New York mid-summer day, not too hot but still comfortable. As we approached mid-block we met a young lady who I had seen years before at the house where she lived. At that time she was a girl of fourteen with long braids down her back.
>
> The girl I set my eyes on now was the most beautiful person I had ever seen—large, soft, warm brown eyes, a glowing color in her dimpled cheek, a cleft chin. . . .

(At this point in Jack's reading, his wife, in embarrassment, left the room. The group laughed and Jack continued reading.)

> When we stopped to speak to her she responded in a deep, warm voice. She wore a fox fur round her neck. I couldn't understand why she was dressed like that on such a warm day. The answer was that that day was her birthday and the fur a gift from her aunt. I did not know then of her foible for wearing any new article of apparel regardless of the time of year.

Mrs. Schwartz returned to the group in time to read her own story.

For Lydia Muncy, a retired school teacher, writing is a means of "keeping my mind vigorously active. Several times of late I have been in groups where there has been group singing—singing of songs with which I was very familiar. Much to my dismay I found it very hard to join in the singing. Somehow I could not find the right notes. Singing has always been a happy part of my life. When alone I used to sing at my work, and in school, when the going was hard and the children restless, I frequently started a favorite song. None of this have I done of late. I seem to have lost this precious ability and it's frightening. Writing forced me to recall experiences, to evaluate their importance to me, or someone who might read what I write. I must seek out vital words and phrases and refrain from outworn modes of expressing myself. Spelling and punctuation must be reviewed."

In some cases people have been brought into the group because it seemed to provide the kind of setting in which a person who is depressed or isolated can both feel comfortable and have a sense of achievement. As Wilbur the Pig said of Charlotte the Spider, "It is not often someone comes along who is a true friend and a good writer."

There are two people in the group who are legally blind. They either type or have their pieces typed, and one of us reads them aloud. If she hasn't been able to write that week, one of these women will often say when it's her turn, "Something ____ said reminded me . . ." and she'll go on to talk about her friend's child who hated peas and carrots, or about a slightly risqué story she recalls. One man—who is not really a member of the group, because he is almost completely deaf—was encouraged to write for therapeutic reasons and joins the group only to give readings. Writing has established a new pattern of communication for him. When his work is printed in the local news-paper, old friends write to him and readers send him their own memories, awakened by his articles.

Whether the motivation for joining a writing group comes from external or internal reasons, the mystery of why people write is everpresent. Mary Grindstaff pinpoints this enigma neatly: "Why do I write? Can you tell me why or how a robin builds a nest or why or how a dog will return home even though it may take weeks or months to get there? Why does a farmer farm? Why does a cotton stalk grow bolls of cotton instead of cockle burr or a stalk of corn grow corn instead of tomatoes? Don't you think it may be the kind of stuff we are made out of, the mold in which we were cast? Don't you think we were made by someone who had something to do with it—the same as why do you like to sing and why you can sing?"

Structure and Format

Both groups meet weekly all year long, with an occasional week or two off. The continuity has been important since it allows members to be absent when ill or on vacation yet return to the group and be welcomed. During long absences group members visit the absentee or write or telephone him. Very few have left the group permanently. The awareness that the group is there, to return to after a long illness, has been important for individual members.

In the beginning we established the pattern of having each person read for five to ten minutes, followed by group discussion to criticize the writing. Whether the material read is criticized from a literary standpoint or not is generally determined by the reader. Some request it; others don't like it. The group discussion is considered by most of the members to be as important as the writing. It is in the discussion that moral points are debated, scraps of history traded, and forgotten stories remembered. The interchange may be heated. It is more often polite. The presence of people with strong religious beliefs, others with doubts, and conservative Republicans and Socialists created tension at times, but the group gradually developed a norm of extreme tolerance. One can disagree but not offend.

At the first session the group requested weekly assignments. Borrowing topics from Koch and Kaminsky, and usually adopting a chronological view of life, my first assignments were:

1. When my Parents Were Young.
2. Bring a photo of yourself as a child and write about it in the first person.
3. Bring a photo of school days and write about it in the third person.
4. Describe a "one word feeling" without using that word—either real or fictional.
5. Early Teens.
6. An Awakening.
7. What others thought of you when you were in your twenties.
8. Something I never told anyone.
9. Marriage.

Several points soon became clear. First, people wanted assignments in order to have something to write about if they got stuck, and to have an opportunity to demonstrate independence from me, the leader. We have had extended periods without assignments, but people invariably ask for them. Sometimes the assignment is suggested by a member of the group. As the group developed, most people knew what they wanted to do and undertook their own projects. An assignment often provided an escape from a long-term project or tickled someone's fancy leading to a new area of exploration.

Second, a time-frame located strictly in the past would not be possible. We jumped from past to present. The first 20 minutes of each session were usually devoted to what had happened to the members during the week and lead us in many directions. After a time people began looking at the clock—it's time for the reading to begin. Third, beginning with one's family history encouraged intimacy and influenced the subsequent feeling that the group itself was a family. "I've told you things I've never told anyone else," a group member said once. When one man wrote about a woman he had loved when he was twenty—a woman who had rejected him for reasons he still did not understand—there was a feeling we all had of being entrusted with the privilege of his confidence. When he cried, so did some of us, and as the group went over the circumstances, trying to find a clue for her behavior, suggesting alternate approaches he could have taken, the whole moment became immediate: He was twenty again and we were now back there with him. We knew this man had been happily married for many years, but our reliving the past with him offered comfort and reassurance, and revealed our mutual puzzlement.

Lastly, sharing each other's writing led to sharing tangible proof that what was being written was indeed true. One week we heard the end of Mary Haynes Grindstaff's story of herself as a young girl on her family's farm, and how she shot a mad dog:

> I climbed the three gates and the fence to make sure the fence was between me and the dog. Would he still be there? If he was not what would I do? Yes, there he sat, in the same spot, in the same way, facing toward me—the same tortured and painful look in his blurry eyes.
>
> I stopped in a good position and resting the gun on my left hand against a post, I threw the safety catch, pressed the gun tight to my shoulder, took a good steady aim and gently pulled the trigger. There was no sound except the gun. There was no movement except that of the dead dog as the forepart of its body fell to the earth.
>
> Oh, poor, poor dog. I threw the empty shell away and reloaded the gun with the spare bullet, put on the safety and walked toward home. At the front yard gate my parents were waiting, papa with a shovel and mother weeping softly. I took her hand and we walked across the bare front yard to the house where I replaced the gun. I had done what I must, what I must. There were the noon dishes to do.

The next week Mary brought in a coke bottle cap with a perfect hole in the middle, ultimate proof of her expertise in shooting a rifle. Less dramatic items such as photographs, souvenirs, and postcards from trips, wild flowers, and books are often shared as each object takes on renewed meaning.

Themes

The themes which emerged from the group are the themes of life—work, friendship, love, childhood, death, nature, parents and children, children and teachers, changing values in society, the mysteries of human behavior. Both the writing and the discussion about the writing serve as a reassessment of the experiences and the judgments once made about them. Time becomes fluid in several ways. In one session, going from writer to writer, we hear about childhood, young parenthood, great grandmothers, and the death of Sadat. But it is primarily in the work of each writer that we understand how stages of life do not end neatly; how events in one period reappear in another. Solutions once made, judgments once arrived at are reexamined in the light of present experience. When this process becomes a group activity, it is as though data from conflicting sources were illuminating one incident thereby forcing the writer to reinterpret it and the other group members to reexamine similar experiences of their own.

For example, one man wrote about a time when both he and his friend were in their twenties. The writer had introduced his friend to a woman from a family with whom he had a close relationship. His friend and the woman fell in love and decided to marry. The writer's dilemma was: should he tell the woman and her family that his friend had been committed to a mental institution several years before, or should he remain quiet? His decision was not to tell the family. The couple married, had a child, and, after a few years, the man's illness returned. His wife went through harrowing times, recounted in the story, and her husband eventually returned to a mental hospital where he died. The story was untitled. One group member suggested it be called, "An Ethical Dilemma." The group debated the writer's decision. Some felt he should have warned the woman before marriage, others felt he had acted properly. In the course of the discussion the group discussed their attitudes about insanity and how these had changed through the years, how their own feelings about "craziness" had changed. In this instance, the resolution achieved seemed to be that the writer should cease to worry about his decision; a child had come out of the marriage and something good had indeed occurred.

Memories are selective and some people, more than others, choose not to write about painful experiences. But each member, as he becomes comfortable, moves from the neutral and abstract to the more personal. And each has a different way of expressing this move. A man who started speaking English at the age of 45 writes:

As far as I can remember I used to tell myself stories—or worse, they used to tell them to me themselves. Of these I have a huge collection, and I am afraid I shall never write down even a fraction, ever. That's why I never liked to chronicle part or all of my life—which, by the way, was just too full of events. I write because I love to write and because I am terribly curious about what will come out.

Groups such as these must respond to the fluidity of life, for although these people have lived full lives, their lives are not static and the process of writing is an evolving one, which takes place very much in the present. Leon Edel writes, "There is evidence that creation is a work of health and not of illness, a force for life."[16] The excitement of these groups lies in reviewing lives over an extended time span, and in watching those lives unfold, still being created right in front of us.

Values

One group opened with Toni Hermann exclaiming: "I heard a song on the radio just before I came here—Frank Sinatra—and I was never so horrified. The song was "I'll do it my way." What is this business, I'll do it my way? What about doing it somebody else's way?"

Changing values in society are often discussed without agreement. The Depression was not the same for everyone. People have different expectations for their children, and former teachers do not agree that schools or children were better then. Frances Lombard recounted for us the lives of people she knew in a small lumbering town in Northern Michigan. In one story, an old Italian woman is forced to deed her house to her son when her husband dies and, eventually, finds herself without a place to live. The wife of the president of the lumber company gathered the immigrant children of the laborers in her house at Christmas to hand out presents in an atmosphere of warm and glittering luxury. Frances weaves fiction and fact together to give us a picture of the town at one critical point in time. We hear later how it has changed and how she is remembered. She returns for a visit and meets her old students who give her a party and celebrate her life as a teacher—giving her even new memories about which to write.

Teaching in a rural school, for example, Lydia Muncy helped the children devise a plan to clean the toilets without embarrassing the little boy who didn't always reach the toilet in time. The values in work, religion, and community are charted and sometimes judgments are made as to whether or not things are better now. But the diversity of opinions and backgrounds creates a complex tapestry so that recognition of present values and how they have changed becomes an ongoing process.

The potential for change each person has within himself is another frequent theme. Agnes Fries's poem is a favorite for its concise statement of this theme:

Never Say Never

"I will n-e-v-e-r go to Japan," she said
　But circumstances forced her to go,
　And she loved it.

"N-e-v-e-r give me eggplant to eat because I hate it," she said,
　But they gave her that Greek dish called moussaka,
　And she loved it.

"I will n-e-v-e-r eat a bite of squid," she said,
　But after that first taste,
　She loved it.

"N-e-v-e-r give me any of those Roman classics to read," she said,
　But Charlie gave her a copy of Herodotus,
　And she loved it.

"N-e-v-e-r ask me to write memoirs of family history," she said,
　But she joined a group doing just that,
　And she loved it.

N-e-v-e-r say n-e-v-e-r," she finally learned.

The following selections illustrate some of these themes. (Although most of the writing is prose, poetry is overrepresented here for the sake of brevity.)

On reading a book, *Mothers and Daughters* by Nancy Friday, "a book that is like surgery for me," Antonie Hermann writes:

Reflection After Reading a Book

I washed the window of my soul
With tears of guilt and sorrow.
It instantly revealed my plight.
Seeing clearly stopped my flight,
But left the promise of tomorrow mirrored.

"Mine is a very simple faith. I find God in nature, in the beauty of people and things. God is goodness and love. I find him in my church. Attendance there is about the only regular thing in my life. It gives order to my days. . . ." (Ardith King).

In the following excerpt the young Agnes Fries is at a revival meeting, thinking about the various sins in her life—damaging her cousin's bike, coming home late. She hears the evangelist ask:

"Will those of you who stood and confessed that your life was not all it should be please come down here in front of the altar?" Woe, woe, alas. This Margaret had not anticipated. It was the farthest thing from her mind, but having committed herself thus far she felt obliged to follow through, so she bravely walked down the steps from that seat high up in the sixth row, trembling with embarrassment all the way, around to the front of the altar with the other twenty-five or thirty people who had appeared there. Many of those on their feet had sat down again, but this possibility had not occurred to Margaret. She had walked the "sawdust trail."

There was nothing offensive or difficult about the next few minutes. She began to understand that she had not really been expected there, that the invitation was for "real sinning" adults. Margaret never forgave the church for exposing her to this ordeal. She never felt the same about religion again. She felt injured.

Isle Royale

There is an island that I love,
    Where peace and quiet reign.
Nothing but blue skies above.
    No hint of hate or pain.

Wildflowers blossom undisturbed,
    Birds sing in the trees,
Little animals unperturbed
    Roam where 'ere they please.

The lake lies peaceful all around
    But when the wind is blowing,
White caps make a hissing sound
    Small boats to shore are rowing.

At twilight high in yonder pine
    The lovely white-throat sings;
Oh! heavenly bird, these notes of thine
    A happy memory brings.

A moose wades in a quiet lake,
  As evening mists close in
He lifts his head—the aspens quake
  As the crickets start to sing.

Oh! royal isle, remote and free
  Your charms have won my heart
Someday I'll journey back to thee
  And per-chance 'ere depart.

Adelaide H. Karsian

Ode to a New Grandson

At evening when the sun has set
  And darkness draws its curtain o'er the day.
Splendid the firmament that sparkles in the night
  And stillness gently comes as noises steal away.

When e'er a door is opened, whenever a babe is born,
  There lies ahead a pathway with promise for everyone.
How like the babe in the manger, two thousand years ago,
  You bring the joy of heaven to those who love you so.

Unsullied by the dusty road, the cares that weigh us down,
  We see in you the goals attained that man has never found.
The stars, those chariots in the sky, they beckon you to rise
  Above the plodding crowd and lead mankind on high.

We know not what may lie ahead, your life has just begun,
  But what we have in mind for you is shining like the sun.
And so dear one, the youngest on our tree,
  We place in you our only hope of immortality.

Lewis B. Kellum

Widow

The first night alone
How wide the bed
The first night alone
On the pillow
Only my head
The first night alone.

Ardith King

I Remember—Oh, I Remember

The palms of my hands remember the shape of your face as they once cupped it.
My thumbs remember the bristles of your heavy brows as they once stroked them.
My fore fingers remember the shape of your straight nose as they once smoothed it.
My third fingers remember the feel of your firm chin as they once came together around it and marked its cleft.
My fourth fingers remember the shape of your lips as they once traced their curves.
My arms remember the strength of your neck as they once clasped it.
My ears remember the sharp, short escape of your breath as you held me quickly and close.
My body remembers the feel of your hard body as we pressed together.
My heart remembers—that you have gone.

Frances Lombard

Birthday

I expect too much of him,
I thought
He's really just a child.
How could he remember?
How could he recall?
It's really nothing much at all.
Yet my heart yearned,
My stomach churned,
Knowing he'd forgotten.

Ardith King

Writing and aging, then, have special significance. They enhance each other. And for the younger person who participates, they can alter his conception of his own life process. I feel as though I now have a longer view; what is happening to me now will likely come up again sometime later. What will I think of it then?

A 77-year-old Japanese woman beautifully captures the effects that writing can have:

I make a paper airplane
With an old calendar

And sail it through the air
Sending off those by-gone days,
Along with bitter memories.

Kumatani Choki (Translated by William F. Sibley)

Notes

[1]G. Berg, & S. Gadow, "Toward More Human Meanings of Aging: Ideals and Images from Philosophy and Art," in S. Spicker, K. Woodward, and D. Van Tassel, (eds.), *Aging and the Elderly: Humanistic Perspectives in Gerontology* (Atlantic Highlands, NJ: Humanities Press, 1978).

[2]L. Edel, *Henry James—The Treacherous Years: 1895–1901* (Philadelphia: J. B. Lippincott, 1969).

[3]M. Kaminsky, *What's Inside You, It Shines Out of You* (New York: Horizon Press, 1974).

[4]M. Kaminsky, "What's Inside You, It Shines Out of You," in R. Gross, B. Gross, and S. Seidman, (eds.), *The New Old* (Garden City, NY: Anchor Books, 1978).

[5]Alvarez, J., & P. Oldham, *Old Age Ain't for Sissies* (Cameron, North Carolina: Crane's Creek Press, 1979).
Bloom, J., "A Window Was Opened to Me," *Teachers & Writers* 12:1(1980): 15–22.
Koch, K. *I Never Told Anybody* (New York: Random House, 1977).
Wolfe, L. "A Kind of Odyssey," *Teachers & Writers* 12:1(1980): 27–32.

[6]P. Cahill, *The Arts, The Humanities and Older Americans* (Washington, D.C., The National Council on Aging, 1981).

[7]P. Campbell, "Report on Arts and Humanities Cultural Forums," *The Arts, The Humanities and Older Americans* (Washington, D.C., The National Council on Aging, 1981).

[8]E. Erikson, & J. Erikson, "Introduction: Reflections on Aging," in S. Spicker, K. Woodward and D. Van Tassel, (eds.), *Aging and the Elderly: Humanistic Perspectives in Gerontology* (Atlantic Highlands, NJ: Humanities Press, 1978).

[9]B. Meyerhoff, & V. Tufte, "Life History as Integration: An Essay on an Experimental Model," *The Gerontologist* 15 (1975):541–543.

[10]B. Meyerhoff, *Number Our Days* (New York: E. P. Dutton, 1978).

[11] M. LoGerfo, "Three Ways of Reminiscence in Theory and Practice,"*International Journal of Aging and Human Development* 12:1 (1980–81):39–47.

[12]V. Revere, & S. Tobin, "Myth and Reality: The Older Person's Relationship to His Past," *International Journal of Aging and Human Development* 12:1 (1980–81): 15–26.

[13]R. Blythe, *The View in Winter* (New York: Harcourt, Brace, Jovanovich, 1979).

[14]I. Progoff, *At a Journal Workshop* (New York: Dialogue House Library, 1975).

[15]The lack of formal education is true of several members of the group who had to leave school for economic reasons early in their lives. However, their keen awareness and disappointment over not being able to continue in school was accompanied by a lifelong, deliberate self-education. Therefore, the barriers between them and those in the group with advanced degrees are nonexistent. One woman, who customarily prefaces her work with an apology for her lack of "book learning," is generally shouted down by the group. This heterogeneity of background contributes to the variety and breadth of the writing; it is a characteristic the group members find highly agreeable.

[16]L. Edel, *Henry James—The Treacherous Years: 1895–1901*.

PART IV
DESIGNING AND DISABILITY

13

Advocacy Design in the Nursing Home: Cultivating Public and Private Spaces for the Newly Admitted Resident

RUTH STUMPE BRENT

Introduction

A nursing home is the dwelling for all who are living there. Too often this dwelling fails to provide a humane and supportive setting that encourages a creative, enriching life style. "Advocacy design" in the institutional setting is an effort to achieve humane and supportive environments for residents of institutions who are unable to assert their own needs. It is time to sensitize health care providers to the complexities of physical environments and to advocate good design for the institutionalized elderly whether they be slightly or severely disabled.

A designer relies upon many available resources including manufacturers' catalogues and specifications for health care furnishings; local, state, and federal building code requirements; data on barrier-free design; and literature concentrating on the behavioral aspects of design.[1] Along with these available external resources the designer, facility manager, administrator, medical director, nursing director, rehabilitation consultants, and others must become involved in playing an active role in fact-finding, or "programming," to determine the needs for maintenance, aesthetics, durability, flexibility, affordability, and, most important of all, special needs of the users.

The task of designing a long-term care institution is complicated. To facilitate the problem-solving process it is necessary to involve all participants—especially the resident-user—in the planning. The designer may need to represent the resident user of the institution, thereby functioning as designer advocate. The designer advocate is particularly important for the institutionalized elderly because of their increased need for a supportive environment as expressed in Lawton and Nahemow's "docility hypothesis."[2] That is, as health and competence decline, the elderly become more vulnerable to environmental influences. This chapter briefly outlines some of the important issues which must be addressed by the designer advocate in the nursing home setting and identifies research relevant to institution programming, the first step in the process of design. As a second step in the design process, a design concept is suggested to alleviate the problems of this alien institutional environment for a newly admitted resident. These two topics are examples of the first two stages in the design process as identified by Zeisel.[3]

Programming for a Nursing Home

Design programming captures the desired range of specific human requirements a building must satisfy in order to support and enhance the performance of human activities.[4] It is also the coherent, meaningful compilation of facts needed to create institutions which will link the management of a complex organization and the user of its buildings to the planning, design, and operation of those institutions.[5]

The numerous factors and relevant information about a site are complex and interrelated. Often, these factors are categorized into three classifications—human, physical, and external factors. The actual programming procedures are stated as a pattern of operations as follows:

- Establish project goals
- Organize programming effort
- Investigate issues
- Interpret information
- Instruct designer and client

• Evaluate results
• Recycle information[6]

Before establishing the project goals of a nursing home there may be preliminary exposure to some of the problems, and brainstorming. Then a list of significant human factors, physical factors, and external factors in a nursing home which seem problematic may be developed. An incomplete list of these issues within the human and physical categories to be addressed by the designer advocate is presented in Figure 13–1. Based on such lists, general project goals

FIGURE 13–1. Nursing home design: human and physical factors.

SAFETY (e.g., BARRIER FREE DESIGN)
WINDOWS
FLOOR COVERING, WALL COVERING, WINDOW TREATMENT
FURNISHINGS
PRIVACY
PERSONALIZATION
COMMUNICATION
COMFORT
RESIDENTS' PARTICIPATION IN THE CONTROL OF THEIR ENVIRONMENT
FLEXIBILITY FOR CHANGING NEEDS
PHYSICAL ENVIRONMENT SUPPORTIVE OF MAINTENANCE OF NON-
  INSTITUTIONAL LIFE STYLE
ENVIRONMENTAL ORIENTATION (SIGNAGE, TRAFFIC FLOW, COLOR COD-
  ING, TEXTURAL CODING)
NONVERBAL MESSAGES (STIGMA/CARING, etc.)
TEMPERATURE LEVELS
LIGHTING
ODOR
APPEARANCE OF A HUMANE ENVIRONMENT
  RESIDENT IDENTITY (e.g., NAMES & PHOTOS ON DOORS)
  ORDERLINESS/CLUTTER
  CLEANLINESS
  SEATING ENCOURAGING/DISCOURAGING SOCIAL INTERACTION
    [SOCIOPETAL/SOCIOFUGAL]
  USE OF COLOR & TEXTURES
  STIMULATION LEVEL
  INSTITUTIONAL VS. RESIDENTIAL CHARACTER
THE USE OF PUBLIC SOCIAL SPACES

---

may be identified which can focus on the programming efforts. Two of these project goals which will be illustrated here are the cultivation of public social spaces for newly admitted residents, and the cultivation of private spaces for newly admitted residents.

Programming Project Goal: #1 Cultivating Public Social Spaces for Newly Admitted Residents

As an example of one project goal, consider the use of public social spaces (e.g., lounges, lobbies, corridors, dining and recreation rooms) in a nursing home where elderly can go to fulfill important emotional and social needs for companionship, activities, and relationships with others.

Sometimes novelists provide more convincing and insightful statements of the human condition than are available from social and behavioral research. John Steinbeck writes about a family living in a rural home with a porch. His colorful imagery portrays the porch as a place for tortoise-shell cats; mothers waving an apron in welcome to an approaching visitor; mothers striking the triangle in a call for breakfast; a place where an old man can get some sun; and a restful place where an old man can sit back and drink lemonade with his grandson.[7]

In a study by McAvoy (1979), the needs for leisure participation most frequently identified by the elderly were the needs of socializing and self-fulfillment. The preferred activity most frequently identified in that study was "visiting friends and relatives." These leisure needs and leisure preferences are fulfilled in the use of public social spaces such as porches, streetcorners, and shopping malls for the elderly living in the community.[8]

For the institutionalized elderly, all the socializing and self-fulfillment needs must be met under the single roof of the health care setting. Their "life space" exists exclusively within the confines of the physical walls of the institution. For the institutionalized elderly, the entrance lobby where there are delivery persons, administrators, and visitors coming and going, the lounge space where there is a television and structured activities, and the immediate space surrounding the nursing station take on special significance. These are the institutional public social spaces where they can go to socialize and engage in various activities. Meanwhile, a lounge removed from the core of activity, at the end of a hall—no matter how stylish and physically attractive—is poorly placed and seldom used.

Special attention should be given to the diversity of activities observed in public social spaces in a nursing home. This diversity contributes to the data base of the nursing home "program" and is an important consideration for the eventual design of new or renovated facilities. For example, activities such as watching television and talking on the telephone may be incompatible with one another and therefore should be located in different areas. Knowing the frequencies of these activities provides information about the type of furnishings needed. Perhaps the institution needs fewer geriatric chairs where residents often sit and fall asleep, and more conversational seating which encourages a better posture for informal and confidential discussions with family and friends.

Observations of residents coded on behavioral maps provide useful program data. Physicians frequently recommend that residents walk for exercise. However, attention to the route of one's walk may be revealing. If the design of the facility has a "circuit" and a resident is able to walk around some area, there may be greater willingness to participate in the exercise than if the facility has only one long hall and the resident is simply walking the same path back and forth. Facilities configured in a double stem "T," a circle, or even an "L" where a resident goes outdoors to complete the circuit, are to be preferred to the common double loaded "Straight Line" corridor (see Figure 13-2).

The corridor, as an important public social space, contributes significantly to the assimilation of a new resident to a nursing home. Within corridors, accessories such as the following, are visible: bulletin boards, birthday boards, signs, mirrors, announcements, newsclip boards, snapshots from special activities, photographs of staff, photographs of residents and their room numbers, drinking fountains, telephones, handrails, and door decorations. These individualized rooms give identity and orientation to residents, create a caring appearance, communicate a friendly social environment on the part of the institution, and may encourage independence and activity.

When a nursing home is under scrutiny and a replacement or renovation is being programmed, the existing institution may be investigated with a combination of methods: participant and nonparticipant observations, questionnaire interviews of all participants (management, staff, residents, and visitors), photography, behavioral maps, and other research techniques. Other sources of program-

FIGURE 13–2. Design configurations and walking circuits.

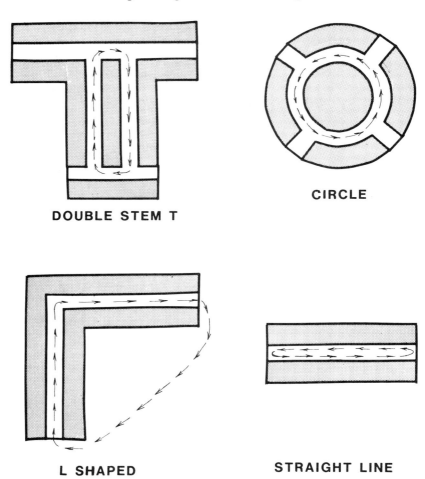

DOUBLE STEM T

CIRCLE

L SHAPED

STRAIGHT LINE

ming information might include observations of similar facilities, drawings and programs of other nursing homes, codes and mandatory requirements, and past research reported in the literature in the areas of environmental psychology, interior design, architecture, gerontology, and other studies of environment and behavior.

Research employing these techniques often reveals problems such as infrequently used lounges with accessibility problems for wheelchair residents; seating arrangements which inadvertently encourage ("sociopetal") or discourage ("sociofugal") conversation; glare from windows which distorts vision; signs with color combinations difficult to distinguish due to the natural yellowing of the eye with age; unsafe flooring in the facilities; and other problems. Based on these problems, program recommendations are developed. The program is the culmination of research in the form of a document stating the requirements of the client/users and the needs of the project for design. The programming process leads to the strengthening of design advocacy for the elderly user.

Programming Project Goal: #2 Cultivating the Private Space for the Newly Admitted Resident

Despite the good intentions of staff, administrators, and designers, the nursing home institutional environment is an alien replacement of residents' former living arrangements. In some rural nursing homes it is not an uncommon circumstance for newly admitted elderly to ride an elevator for the first time in their lives to reach their small semiprivate room. As the nurse inquires how many blocks the newly admitted resident can walk, the rural elderly individual must convert cornfield distances to city block distances.

As Lawton points out in his book, *Environment and Aging,* "the dwelling unit is where individuality may be maximally expressed; the disruption of such a long-term expression of the self by moving or going to an institution may be a major trauma."[9] The detrimental effects of institutionalization on older people has been more fully articulated by the Ebenezer Center for Aging (Minneapolis, Mn.) as:

An institution is not "home."
Relocation may have a negative effect on health and even cause death.
Nursing home residents are segregated from people of other ages and from friends and family members.
Entering an institution makes some people feel rejected.
Entering an institution represents a loss of status.
Living in an institution causes loss of independence.
Living in a nursing home symbolizes approaching death.
There is a loss of former roles.
There is a loss of control over one's life.
There is limited opportunity for choices.
There is a lack of privacy.
Needs for territoriality may be thwarted.

Institutions foster dependence.
Residents may lose function.
Institutions sometime foster maladaptive behavior.[10]

Making the transition from the home situation to a nursing home or other institution for long-term care is frequently difficult. Allowing a person to take at least one particularly meaningful piece of furniture and other "treasures" helps to alleviate the dramatic change of home environments. There is an effort in many nursing homes to encourage room personalization. This personalization contributes to a resident's feeling of belonging and permits expressions of "territoriality." Elderly persons living in their own homes are surrounded by a wealth of plants, pictures, candles, coffee table display pieces, bedroom chests, boxes, bottles, and memorabilia. The vast array of accessories reflect the personalities and experiences of the individuals who live there. Objects serve as symbols of continuity.

Expressions of uniqueness and individuality in the nursing home setting are apparent in how residents mark or "flag" their territority. Ribbons, wreaths, and colored paper by names on private room doors are frequently used to distinguish their own door from the many others along a long corridor. In semiprivate rooms, wall spaces display photographs, calendars, bows, craft items, plants, and collections. Geriatric chairs and wheelchairs are adapted with pillows, fur skins, and pouches for comfort, function, and individual appeal.[11] In complete contrast to the proliferation of these items, some long-term care institutions are devoid of personal expressions. The walls and furniture tops are barren and the most private spaces in semiprivate rooms are limited to the territory of one's own bed.

In a study of the effect of the presence of personal belongings on perceptions of the elderly in institutions, two groups of medical students were asked their impressions of the same elderly person. For one group, the elderly person was surrounded by personal belongings. For the second, the setting was bare. The elderly person surrounded by personal belongings was perceived in a less negative way than the same person in bare surroundings. The authors note that the patients are likely to benefit by having some "non-hospital environment" around themselves and "at the very least, this gives doctors something else to talk about besides the resident's condition (And how are we today?) and the weather."[12]

A person recently admitted into a nursing home tends to be more anxious and requires a more subtle, less demanding, and less arousing environment than someone who has lived there a longer period of time.[13]

As Tobin and Lieberman write in *Last Home for the Aged,* when elderly are newly admitted to an institution there is an "immediate reaction, often taking the form of extreme confusion or severe with-drawal, which slowly subsides as the elderly person adjusts to the demands of the setting."[14] The authors explain that the person goes through a series of phases in adjustment and assimilation within the nursing home. The second phase, occurring after the immediate entrance phase, is an initial adjustment phase which takes place within the first two months after entering the home. The third phase lasts until the end of the first year. At the end of phase three, the resident "has either adapted to the institution and survived intact or has deteriorated or died."[15] These difficult transition phases may be eased by an institutional environment designed to provide extra support to new residents to smooth their transition. For example, the room of the newly admitted resident may be less stimulating in color and pattern and more residential in feeling with accommodations for photographs and memorabilia.

Closely related to the importance of possessions to a newly admitted resident are the spatial-behavioral issues of personal space, privacy, territoriality, and general control of one's near environment. Alton DeLong has noted the age changes in sensory perception and spatial aspects of communication.[16]

Because vision, hearing, touch, and smell all decline with age, spatial behavior also varied with age. Younger institutional staff members felt their personal space had been invaded by elderly who wanted to move close enough to touch, hear, and see them.

Territoriality—the phenomenon of turf protection—and privacy have been reported on in the classic work of Goffman.[17] Goffman's work in mental institutions examined the lack of control residents have over their personal selves, clothing, and possessions. Private possessions were taken away from residents, their bodies were ex-amined at any time, and there were few, if any, private places where they could go to retreat. These findings are depressing reminders of a situation without advocacy design and user-orientation. The issues of spatial behavior are important considerations in the planning of long-term care facilities.

Color contributes both functionally, aesthetically, and psycholo-gically to a health care facility with immediate effect on a new resident. Color may be used to code and give orientation to a long hallway, define objects in space so that one does not trip over furni-ture, and give a feeling of warmth to an otherwise cold, sterile environment. As the least expensive design tool to work with, it

elicits the greatest human response. It is also culturally and personally specific.[18] For example, some ethnic groups prefer more brilliant
colors than others and some individuals enjoy purple while others do
not.

Although the impact of color is a topic of continuing study by
health care designers, some research has indicated that warm and
luminous colors such as the yellows, reds, and oranges tend to induce
increased activity and alertness and are conducive to muscular effort,
action, and a cheerful feeling (Aranyi and Goldman, 1980). Traditionally, cool colors such as pastel blues, violets, and greens are
thought to be calming and passive. The properties of color being hue
(the color itself), value (how much black or white is added to the
color), and intensity (how bright or dull the color is) need to be
carefully controlled. Also, the amount and location of those colors
must be carefully controlled to produce the predicted effect on behavior. For example, a highly saturated bright and vibrant "hot red"
may also be viewed as angry and tension producing.[19] Low intensity
and pastel warm hues (e.g., yellow, gold, peach, etc.), rather than a
bright red, yellow, or orange, may be better color selections for a
newly admitted person; it creates a cheerful, friendly, and calm,
supportive environment without overstimulating an already anxious
resident. However, control of color must be exerted because color
perception may be influenced by other adjacent colors (e.g., other
surfaces and flesh tones of a patient), lighting (e.g., natural light and
lamps), and the quantity of that color (e.g., how many walls are
painted that color).

The Problem and Concept Statement

Information obtained from programming provides the basis for the
"problem statement." The overall product of programming is the
statement of the problem. This problem statement is the last step in
the programming process and the first step in problem solving. It is
this problem statement that provides the premises for design, and
later provides design criteria to evaluate the design solution.[20] Figure 13–3 illustrates a possible problem statement for a nursing
home environment.

After programming has provided a basis for creating a problem
statement, the designer must carry the process to the next step to
develop specific and detailed design recommendations. These specific

FIGURE 13–3. Problem statements.

The nursing home tends to be an alien environment for most elderly and there is great need to provide public social spaces where residents can fulfill their emotional and social support needs in an attempt to maintain their former noninstitutional life style. With the significance of these needs, the physical design of the public social spaces should give special attention to resident individuality, support for privacy, as well as socialization and orientation.

Because the design configuration of corridors within a nursing home may have a positive effect upon the walking patterns of elderly and because physicians encourage walking as exercise, the corridor configuration should be a "circuit" without requiring the resident to walk outside of the building in inclement weather.

Because the newly admitted resident is highly anxious and requires a low stimulus near-environment and because the new resident has difficulty personally in making the transition from a private residential location to a public institution, a "Transition Room" is suggested which has more privacy than the typical semiprivate room, has a more residential and less institutional character, and accommodates a high degree of personalization.

---

recommendations are called "concept statements" and they should, so far as possible, provide design solutions to the problems posed by the problem statement. Figure 13–4 and 13–5 illustrate the design concept statements for nursing home public social spaces and the recommended private space called a "Transition Room." Figures 13–6 and 13–7 further illustrate potential designs based upon these concepts. Figure 13–6 is a floor plan and Figure 13–7 is an elevation drawing of a standard semiprivate-sized room adapted as a private "Transition Room." This design concept is specifically geared to advocacy design for the newly admitted resident.

Summarizing the Design Process and Facilities Planning

The philosophy of "advocacy design" is a continuing, user-oriented process in which the needs and desires of all users of the space are determined by research, and communicated and articulated in the form of a design concept. The facility is constructed, and its use and adaptation is followed by postoccupancy evaluation of the environment.[21] This approach requires the participation of diverse interest groups as well as teamwork to balance and unify decision making. The design advocacy procedure in a nursing home setting strives to achieve good design that is humane and supportive.

Often "good design" costs no more than "bad design." The choice of one color over another costs the same and the selection of appropriate furnishings which may originally cost more may be less expensive when considered over the entire life cycle.

There are, of course, limits to what can be achieved by changes made to the physical environment. However, the benefits of "good design" are difficult to measure quantitatively. Irwin Altman's environment-behavior theory suggests that environment and behavior

FIGURE 13–4.   Concept statements: Public social spaces.

—Located near service, delivery, and entrance areas
—Located near nursing station
—Located near any other social activity area (busy sidewalks, children's playground, etc.)
—Seating accommodations for conversational groupings (sociopetal)
—Seating accommodations for watching television
—Television placement at seated eye level (not hung from ceiling)
—Windows allowing natural light without glare
—Texture variations in wall coverings and other surfaces
—Warm, medium-intensity contrasting colors to give orientation (color coding hallways, handrails, and information boards; color differentiation for wall and floor planes and figure-ground relationships for differentiation of furnishings and floorspace)
—Well-lit hallways using warm fluorescent lamps and fluorescent luminaires for general lighting
—Supplemental decorative luminaires to add residential character (e.g., lamps in lounges, chandeliers in dining areas)
—Convenient bathrooms to encourage use by those concerned with incontinence (located near all lounges, dining room, entrance, and periodically along circuits of travel)
—Corridor accessories to provide a more personal character and give orientation (signage, full length mirrors, clocks, calendars, newspaper clipping boards, birthday boards, photographs and names of residents, photographs and names of staff, snapshot photographs taken at special activities, event board, artwork depicting scenes that residents can relate to—such as pastoral scenery or still-life of food,—drinking fountain, telephone located in a private nook where residents can sit down, and magazine racks)

FIGURE 13–4. (*continued*)

—Continuous handrails in corridors

—Accessories should be placed at standing eye level and below—for wheelchair residents to comfortably read and enjoy them

—Accessories should be selected with color hue and value contrast to facilitate reading (e.g., because of the natural yellowing of one's eyes, an elderly person cannot distinguish certain greens and blues). White letters on black background has good contrast for readability.

—Vinyl upholstery fabric on chairs that can be used by incontinent residents but that may have a visual texture or pattern to seem less institutional

—Lounges providing different types of seating than all geriatric chairs

—Seating arrangements in clusters—not chairs lined up against all the walls

—Window treatment giving a softening effect and more residential in character

—Window treatment filtering or controlling direct sunlight

—Window treatment giving texture and pattern to otherwise slick and plain environments

—Window treatment that is changed seasonally in lounges and dining spaces—to give residents a sense of time and rejuvenation

—Use of laminated wood rather than metal in furnishings to decrease institutional feeling

—Wall coverings that are cleanable yet add texture and interest accenting some spaces (e.g., vinyl wall covering used in entrances and in nursing station area)

—Significant focal points in each area (e.g., fireplace in lounges, plants, scenic murals in dining room, waterfall or fountain, weavings, paintings, sculpture)

—Floor covering that is smooth without being slick: easy to walk on as well as easy for wheelchair use; continuous plane without distracting light or design patterns that seem like objects

---

are closely linked almost to the point of being inseparable. The two are a dynamic system with mutual and dual impact between both people and environments.[22] Accordingly, to become an advocate for the long-term care resident therefore requires advocacy design of the health care environment.

The steps in the design process illustrated here for the new resident in the nursing home are only the first of many. Responsible design does not end with the concept, but provides a continuing basis for feedback and communication with facility users. This includes postoccupancy evaluations and effects to adjust the physical design features of the environment as users respond to the changes and as new problems become evident. Recognition of this dynamic, evolving, and continuing need for modification and adaptation of the environ-

FIGURE 13–5. Concept statements: Transition room for the newly admitted resident.

—Located near the central area of activity, not isolated at the end of a hall
—Located near a social area such as a lounge or dining room
—Seating accommodations for conversation without having to use bed
—Windows allowing natural light without glare
—Texture variations in wall coverings and other surfaces
—Pastel colors
—Adequate lighting for reading and dressing area
—Supplemental incandescent lighting that gives more natural and residential character
—Some decorative and noninstitutional lighting fixtures
—Adjacent bathroom with safety and barrier-free requirements
—Provisions for personal photographs, a special chest or chair from the resident's former home, and other small mementos
—Bulletin board for cards and other messages
—Accessories to include clock, calendar, mirror, and framed pictures that an elderly person can relate to
—Colorful bedspread coordinated with window treatment
—Upholstery fabric on chair that can be used by an incontinent resident—and may have a visual texture or pattern
—Window treatment giving a softening effect and more residential in character
—Window treatment filtering and controlling direct sunlight
—Window treatment giving texture but not with a great deal of pattern (pattern, especially large prints, may be too stimulating for newly admitted residents)
—Snap-on, hand-drawn drapery or stationery with stack by wall (these would not have cords that may be dangerous to some mentally disturbed residents). If fabric is tugged on, the drapery would simply come off the rod rather than ripping.
—Variations of bedspreads and coordinated window-treatments available depending upon personal preferences of color
—Use of wood rather than metal in furnishings (chest, seating, bedside table) giving a more residential character
—Chair railing to add a more residential character
—Wallcoverings that are cleanable yet add texture and interest accenting architectural feature of chair railing
—Interesting focal point that resident can enjoy looking at while in bed—for example, outdoor scenery from a window that is low enough to see out while in bed)
—Carpet of a dense, low pile for durability, cleanability, and residential character (Often, fourth generation nylon is recommended.)
—Resident control of temperature in room
—Resident control of open/closed door

FIGURE 13–6. Floor plan.

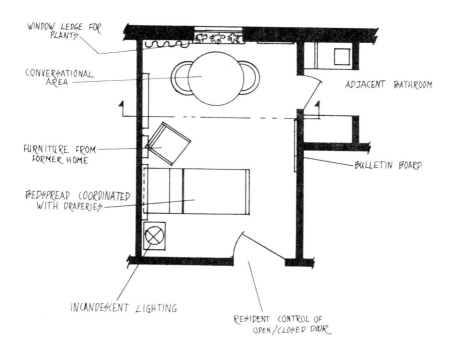

SEMI-PRIVATE ROOM –
CONVERTED TO A "TRANSITION-ROOM"

WINDOW LEDGE FOR PLANTS

CONVERSATIONAL AREA

ADJACENT BATHROOM

FURNITURE FROM FORMER HOME

BULLETIN BOARD

BEDSPREAD COORDINATED WITH DRAPERIES

INCANDESCENT LIGHTING

RESIDENT CONTROL OF OPEN/CLOSED DOOR

174

FIGURE 13-7. Elevation.

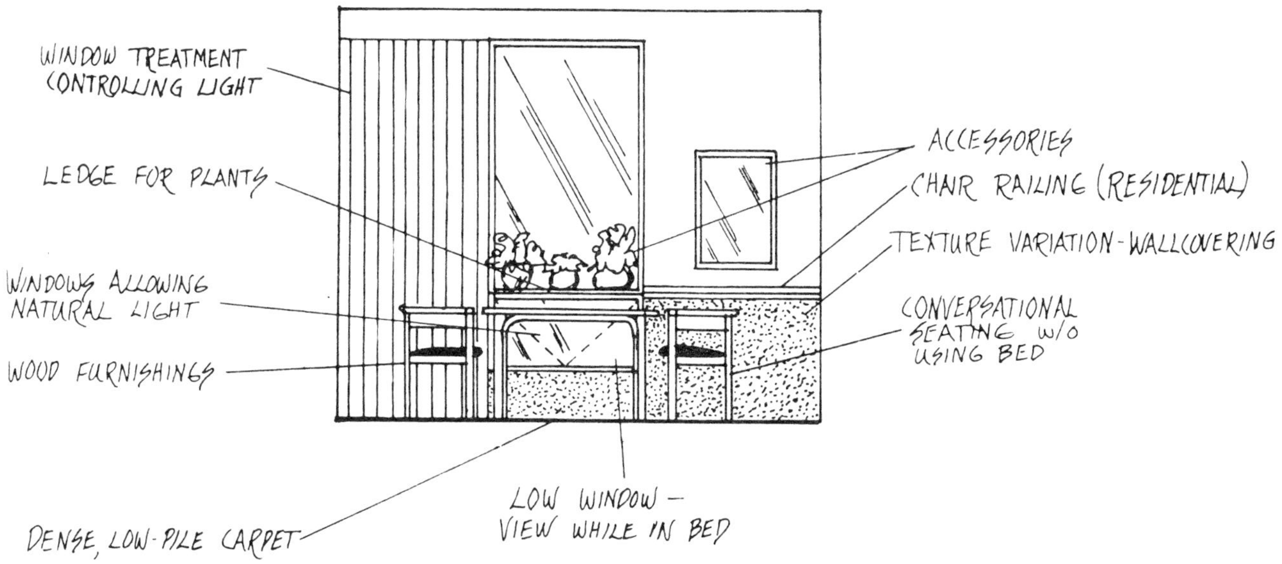

ACCESSORIES

CHAIR RAILING (RESIDENTIAL)

TEXTURE VARIATION - WALLCOVERING

CONVERSATIONAL SEATING W/O USING BED

LOW WINDOW - VIEW WHILE IN BED

WINDOW TREATMENT CONTROLLING LIGHT

LEDGE FOR PLANTS

WINDOWS ALLOWING NATURAL LIGHT

WOOD FURNISHINGS

DENSE, LOW-PILE CARPET

ment throughout its life has led to the development of institutionally-based facilities planners who carry out this work on a continuing basis. To insure advocacy design, a facilities planner is an important participant in the problem-solving team along with an elderly user, interior designer, maintenance personnel, nursing and physician staff, and administration.

Notes

[1]Irwin Altman, *The Environment and Social Behavior: Privacy, Personal Space, Territory, Crowding* (Monterey, CA: Brooks/Cole, 1975).

Aranyi, Laszlo, & Larry L. Goldman, *Design of Long-Term Care Facilities* (New York: Van Nostrand Reinhold, 1980).

Kleeman, Walter B., Jr., *The Challenge of Interior Design* (Boston: CBI Publishing Co. 1981).

Koncelik, Joseph, *Designing the Open Nursing Home* (Stroudsburg, PA: Dowden, Hutchingson and Ross, 1976).

Sommer, Robert, *Personal Space* (Englewood Cliffs, NJ: Prentice-Hall, 1969).

Zeisel, John, *Inquiry By Design: Tools for Environment-Behavior Research* (Monterey, CA: Brooks/Cole, 1981).

[2]M. P. Lawton, & L. Nahemow, "Ecology and the Aging Process," in C. Eisdorfer and M. P. Lawton (eds.), *The Psychology of Adult Development in Aging* (Washington, D.C.: American Psychological Association, 1973).

[3]Zeisel, *Inquiry By Design.*

[4]Michael Brill, *The Architect's Guide to Facility Programming*, Mickey A. Palmer, (ed.) (Washington, D.C.: American Institute of Architects, 1981).

[5]Edward J. Agostini, *The Architect's Guide to Facility Programming*, Mickey A. Palmer (ed.) (Washington, D.C.: American Institute of Architects, 1981).

Davis, Gerald, *The Architect's Guide to Facility Programming*, Mickey A. Palmer (ed.).

[6]Mickey Palmer, *Architect's Guide.*

[7]John Steinbeck, "The Leader of the People," *John Steinbeck: 13 Great Short Stories from the Long Valley* (NY: Avon, 1943).

[8]Ruth Brent, "Community and Institutional Public Social Spaces," *Journal of Therapeutic Recreation*, XVI 1st quarter, 1982, pp. 41–48.

[9]M. Powell Lawton, *Environment and Aging* (Belmont, CA: Brooks/Cole, 1980), p. 62.

[10]Kathy Carroll, ed., *The Nursing Home Environment* (Minneapolis: Ebenezer Center for Aging and Human Development, 1978).

[11]Koncelik, *The Nursing Home Environment.*

[12]P. H. Millard, & C. S. Smith, "Personal Belongings—A Positive Effect?" *The Gerontologist* 21:7 (1981): 90.

[13]Ruth Brent, "Environmental Constraints on the Spatial Organization of Social Interactions in a Nursing Home," HEW HDS-AOA 90 AR 2058 Final Report, University of Missouri, Columbia, Missouri (1981).

Mehrabian, A., *Public Places and Private Spaces* (New York: Basic Books, 1976).

[14]Sheldon S. Tobin, & Morton A. Lieberman, *Last Home for the Aged* (San Francisco: Jossey-Bass, 1978).

[15]——. p. 21.

[16]Alton DeLong, "The Microspatial Structure of the Older Person," in L. A. Pastalan and D. H. Carson (eds.), *The Spatial Behavior of Older People* (Ann Arbor: Institute of Gerontology, University of Michigan, 1970).

[17]Erving Goffman, *Asylums: Essays on the Social Situation of Mental Patients and Other Inmates* (New York: Anchor Books, 1961).

[18]Frank Mahnke, "Color in Medical Facilities," *Interior Design* 52:4 (April, 1981).

[19]Aranyi and Goldman, *Design of Long-Term Care Facilities.*

[20]William Pena, *Problem Seeking: An Architectural Programming Primer* (Boston: Cahners Books International, 1977).

[21]Kleeman, *The Challenge of Interior Design.*

[22]Altman, *The Environment and Social Behavior.*

14

Rehabilitation and the Elderly: Implications for Geriatric Services

RICHARD A. LUSKY

Introduction

Increasing numbers of health professionals—based on practical experience or involvement in geriatric training programs—are moving towards a holistic view of health care for the aged. This does not, however, mean that such care is now being delivered or that it will be easily delivered in the future. I am, of course, referring to the problem of implementing such a model within a system designed for the resolution of acute health problems in otherwise healthy people. I would like to illustrate the nature of these problems with data from a regional study of rehabilitation services in New England.[1] I will argue that it is easier to assemble the resources required by a holistic model of geriatric care than to make the model work. Finally, I will discuss some of the implications of the study for training geriatric health professionals.

Rehabilitation Services in Perspective

The most important feature of contemporary rehabilitation services involves their central and holistic concern with physical and social functioning, rather than cure. This concern has crystalized into a philosophy of care with which many geriatric health professionals identify. Gullickson and Licht, who surveyed the American Congress of Rehabilitation regarding the nature of "rehabilitation medicine," found a strong emphasis on the concept of comprehensive care. Practitioners characterized their activity as the "medical management of disability," noting that such management should be: (1) comprehensive (addressing physical, social, psychological, and vocational limitations), (2) aggressive (rather than a passive response to patient complaints), (3) ongoing (to maintain optimal functioning over time), (4) individualized (to the patient's disability and unique problems), and (5) integrated (with the activities of relevant professionals and the patient's significant others).[2]

A second important feature of contemporary rehabilitation services involves the broad-based support underlying their development. This support extended beyond the health professions. Wesson, observing the heterogeneous sponsorship of rehabilitation services by potential recipients and providers, social service agencies, religious organizations, and philanthropists, has aptly characterized the development of rehabilitation services as a social movement—one whose members sought, and largely obtained, a societal mandate to implement their revolutionary health care philosophy.[3] Straus[4] and Sussman[5] have identified a variety of motives underlying this support, ranging from "humanitarian impulses," to the hope that the rehabilitated would again "pull their own weight" financially.

This broad-based but heterogeneous support led to a third key aspect of contemporary rehabilitation services—their organizational complexity. Rehabilitation's mandate came in the form of progressively increasing but piecemeal federal commitment to the concept. While the first major rehabilitation legislation, enacted in 1918, provided narrowly defined services (vocational retraining) to a narrowly defined population (returning veterans), subsequent legislation extended the scope of services, expanded eligibility criteria, and allocated funds for training rehabilitation personnel, research and development, and new rehabilitation facilities.[6] Medicare and Medicaid, in the mid-1960s, opened the door to the public financing of rehabilitation services following acute hospitalization.[7] Under these legislative stimuli a variety of federal and state facilities and programs were superimposed upon a growing number of disease-specific, impairment-specific, and population-specific rehabilitation programs in the voluntary sector.[8] This expansion was accompanied by the growth of specialized rehabilitation personnel including board-certified physical medicine and rehabilitation specialists, physical and occupational therapists, and rehabilitation nurses among the health professions[9]; and rehabilitation counselors and vocational retraining specialists among the social service professions.[10]

The Study

The study was undertaken to explore the implications of this organizational complexity on the ability of rehabilitation providers to deliver the kind of comprehensive and integrated services associated with the rehabilitation philosophy. To this end, 100 rehabilitation patients from a health planning region rich in rehabilitation resources were interviewed about their "patient careers."[11] The interview data were analyzed to see how regional providers—acting individually, serially, and jointly—actually handled the problems of physical impairment. Where discrepancies between the patients' experiences and the philosophy of comprehensive rehabilitation emerged, these discrepancies were discussed with key rehabilitation providers in the region.

The patients represented four disease/impairment constellations, each of which pose somewhat different rehabilitation challenges. The two "tracer diseases"[12] discussed here, stroke and hip fracture, were selected to illuminate the special rehabilitation problems associated with the aging patient. Both are particularly useful tracers in this regard. Stroke, with an estimated incidence of 20 per 1,000 among those aged 65 to 74, constitutes a major health problem among the elderly which is associated with wide-ranging functional impairment.[13] While its estimated incidence is lower,[14] hip fracture, with its focused trauma, specific impairment, and comparatively straightforward management, is expected to be an increasingly important geriatric health problem for at least three decades.[15] Both problems are the product of underlying chronic disease, are characterized by acute onset, are readily diagnosed, and are typically associated with rapid hospitalization. Despite their overall importance in mortality among the elderly, nearly 80 percent of stroke patients, and nearly 90 percent of hip fracture patients survive the initial acute episode.[16]

In the case of stroke, studies have shown the early initiation of physical therapy to be associated with reduced mortality and improved functioning regardless of the severity of the stroke, the age of the patient, or the presence of concurrent disease,[17] and "post acute" stroke rehabilitation to be associated with functional gains which cannot be attributed to spontaneous recovery.[18] Follow-up data suggest that these functional gains are enduring, and that the costs of rehabilitation are largely offset by decreased rates of rehospitalization. Studies by Muckle,[19] Thomas and Stevens,[20] and Beals[21] show comparable benefits to be associated with early and aggressive rehabilitation for hip fracture patients.

Rehabilitation and the Elderly

While both groups of patients described a variety of problems in the earliest stages of their patient careers (e.g., difficulties in reaching their primary care physicians at onset, problems with transport to the hospital, and delays in admission following diagnosis), I will focus on three problem areas more clearly associated with the rehabilitation process. The first area involves problems encountered in "getting to" community hospital rehabilitation services following admission, and with the "logic of care" once such services are reached. The second problem area involves difficulties with the transition to alternative institutional or community-based programs. The final problem area encompasses discrepancies between the comprehensive rehabilitation model and the actual delivery of "post acute" rehabilitation services in tertiary rehabilitation facilities, long-term care settings, and the community.

Rehabilitation in the Community Hospital

In light of their diverse experiences preceding hospital admission, and their divergent experiences following discharge, initial hospitalization of the stroke and hip fracture patients represented a critical point, organizationally and therapeutically, for initiation of a rehabilitation effort. In most community hospitals this required, as one physiatrist made clear, a referral from the medical floor to an organizationally distinct physical therapy department or rehabilitation unit:

> No patient, regardless of the diagnosis, is transferred to us. We don't have a "physical medicine service" at City Hospital. We don't have our

own patients. We simply work with the patients' physicians on a consulting basis.

(City Hospital Physiatrist)

While most patients did receive at least some physical or occupational therapy during their hospital stay, a fifth of the stroke patients and several hip fracture patients had no formal contact with rehabilitation personnel:

> My mother was given drug treatments. She laid in bed until she was well enough to go home.

(Daughter's recollection)

> I was in bed the whole time I was in the hospital. It took all the strength out of me.

(Patient's recollection)

More important, given the benefits of early rehabilitation, were the delays which characterized many referrals for rehabilitation services. Delaying physical therapy a week or more following the initiation of medical care was common practice, especially with the stroke patients. Delays of two weeks or more were not uncommon:

> My aunt laid in bed for a week. One therapist wanted to start therapy, but the doctor was afraid that something might cause another stroke.

(Niece's recollection)

> I was in the hospital for two weeks. Then they transferred me to a convalescent unit for physical and speech therapy.

(Patient's recollection)

Although some delayed referrals appear to have been tied to the physical separation of rehabilitation services from the medical floors (the rehabilitation unit was typically "downstairs" or "in the next building"), many delays seemed to stem from the admitting and attending physicians' unfamiliarity with rehabilitation concepts and services. In interview, hospital physiatrists confirmed this impression, noting that undergraduate medical students had little exposure to rehabilitation principles, and that residents were unlikely to rotate through rehabilitation departments. The rehabilitation units, functioning as consulting services within the hospital, were dependent on referrals from physicians who knew little about the potential of rehabilitation therapy. Given the semiautonomous character of the medical floors, and the absence of any centralized mechanism for systematic consideration of rehabilitation, physiatrists were forced to rely on the more haphazard vehicles of personal and professional relationships for referrals:

> Referrals to the physical therapy department depend on the relationship between the physiatrist and the attending physicians and residents. I've been here a long while and know a lot of them. I make the rounds on the floors to keep in contact. We get a pretty good number of referrals.

(Catholic Hospital Physiatrist)

It is difficult to accurately assess the therapeutic implications of nonreferrals and delayed referrals to rehabilitation services. It is notable, however, that nearly a third of the stroke patients and half of the hip fracture patients in the study reported developing, while in the hospital, the kinds of secondary complications associated with confinement to bed (decubitus ulcers, contractures, bowel impactions, bladder infections, pneumonia, and emboli).

The organizational and physical isolation of hospital rehabilitation units also had implications for the logic of care provided. Functioning as ancillary services with little or no control over the patient care process, the units were forced to construct rehabilitation schedules around patient care routines established by, and reflecting the needs of, the medical floors. The issue of patient medication illustrates the nature of the problem. In a number of cases, physical therapy was prematurely terminated because the subjects were reportedly "confused" or "uncooperative." While confusion and resistance to therapy might well have been a function of the subject's age or neurologic impairment, the inclusion of hip fracture patients among the terminated cases, and frequent complaints of "over-medication" by both types of patients, suggest difficulties in coordinating medication and rehabilitation schedules:

> They gave me pills in the hospital that were too strong. They made me sleepy all the time so that I couldn't do anything.
>
> *(Patient recollection)*

> Once I got her home, I stopped giving her all those sleeping pills and tranquilizers they had been giving her. And, you know, her mind cleared right up. Before, she didn't know me and wouldn't talk to me. Now she's happy and alert and seems to be quite content.
>
> *(Daughter's recollection)*

Similarly, there was little that rehabilitation personnel could do to ensure that routine patient care complemented the rehabilitation effort. In several instances, in fact, the study's subjects experienced setbacks on the medical floor which might have been avoided in a more structured setting:

> The therapy was going very well and I had learned to use the walker. On the day I was due to be discharged I fell again. I was in the bathroom washing up. When I wanted to use the toilet I rang but no one came. When I started for the door I tripped and the door closed on me. It was half an hour before someone heard me calling. Instead of going home I spent another six weeks in the hospital.
>
> *(Patient recollection)*

> Mother was in the hospital about three months. She would have been out a month earlier but she hurt her back. They said she fell when she tried to get out of bed by herself.
>
> *(Daughter's recollection)*

More important than these "coordination problems" was the effect that separating rehabilitation and ongoing patient care activities had on the overall character of the rehabilitation process. The ability of admitting and attending physicians to bypass rehabilitation personnel and prescribe their own course of physical therapy, and their ultimate control over the timing of hospital discharge (coupled with reimbursement criteria which encouraged the earliest possible discharge) served to undermine the ideals of comprehensive assessment, goal setting, and planning. Few of the patients reported contact with rehabilitation unit physiatrists. Less than half experienced comprehensive evaluation on a rehabilitation unit. While a number of stroke patients received occupational and/or speech therapy, none received any psychological services or other counseling. For the clear majority of the patients the rehabilitation effort was comprised of a more or less routine course of physical therapy designed to "get them on their feet"—a crucial but limited rehabilitation goal in relation to the varied needs of most geriatric patients. In fact, in their almost exclusive concern with ambulation, the hospital rehabilitation departments often prepared the patients to leave the hospital, but failed to prepare them for effective functioning once home:

> They taught me to use a walker in physical therapy. I got around all right when I got home, but I had difficulty getting out of bed and putting on my clothes, and taking a bath.

(Patient recollection)

> I got physical therapy once a day in the hospital. They taught me how to use crutches, but they didn't show me how to get up and down the stairs. When I got home I had to make do as well as I could.

(Patient recollection)

Perhaps the best indication of the extent to which rehabilitation in the community hospital diverged from the comprehensive rehabilitation philosophy was a frequent failure to fully include the patients in the rehabilitation effort:

> Nobody ever told me that I had had a stroke. I don't recall anyone ever telling me exactly what happened. I figured it out myself since I knew people who had had strokes before and I knew the symptoms.

(Patient recollection)

> They didn't tell Dottie all of it for a while because they thought it would be better if she didn't know so she wouldn't worry.

(Niece's recollection)

Discrepancies between the ideals and the realities of comprehensive rehabilitation in the community hospital appear to have been related more to the organizational context in which rehabilitation personnel operated than to declining commitment to the ideals themselves. The comments of the rehabilitation department directors suggest a continuing commitment to the principles of comprehensive rehabilitation, but few practical incentives or opportunities for putting them into practice. In a real sense, the philosophy of acute care, which dominated the community hospital as a whole, had come to dominate rehabilitation efforts as well.

> Ideally, rehabilitation should begin as soon as the patient is stabilized and should attend to all the patient's impairments. The acute care— that's the business of the attending physicans. Then comes the rehabilitation and convalescent care. Getting them to the point where they can do for themselves, that's our job. Ideally, the effort should continue after discharge, and we often recommend that it continue.

> *(City Hospital Physiatrist)*

> Let's face it, the hospital is an acute care facility. We are here to supplement that care. We only have the patients for a short period of time. We try to take them as far as we can during that time. After that, it's up to their doctors and the other programs.

> *(Catholic Hospital Physiatrist)*

Discharge and Predischarge Planning

Approximately one-fourth of the study's stroke patients were independently mobile by the time of their discharge from the community hospital. A third required assistive devices or help from others. The remaining stroke patients were confined to a wheelchair or bed. The hip fracture patients were, as a group, more impaired. None were independently mobile. Nearly two-thirds required assistive devices or help from others, with the remaining third confined to a chair or bed.

Given the limited "acute rehabilitation" goals of the community hospital, relatively few of the patients had reached their optimal level of functioning at discharge. Further rehabilitation efforts, where they were warranted, hinged on an appropriate referral to a rehabilitation facility, long-term care setting with rehabilitation capabilities, or to a community rehabilitation program. Referrals were typically the responsibility of the hospital's social services department when the patient was being transferred to an institutional setting, or a special discharge planning department if the patient was

being returned to the community. Discharge plans from either department required physician approval.

Approximately 80 percent of both groups were, in fact, referred
by the hospital for some type of organized follow-up care. These
referrals were apparently stimulated by the Medicare reimbursement, predischarge planning requirement, designed to ensure that
those elderly who are discharged because they no longer require
acute care will continue to receive needed care at an appropriate
level. Closer examination of referral patterns, however, suggest
several problems in relation to the ideals of comprehensive rehabilitation.

Of the two groups, the stroke patients were the more likely to be
the objects of continuing rehabilitation efforts. Nearly half were
referred to extended care institutions where they were able to receive
at least some therapy, or to rehabilitation hospitals. Most of the
remaining stroke patients were referred to community-based programs offering physical and/or occupational therapy. Despite their
more limited functional status, hip fracture patients were frequently
returned to the community without the benefit of organized services,
or with services limited to nursing care.

Examination of referral patterns in relation to level of impairment showed a number of notable discrepancies in both groups, with
several of the more impaired patients returned to the community
without continuing rehabilitation, and a number of the least impaired patients referred to rehabilitation facilities or community-
based rehabilitation programs. In part, these apparent discrepancies
may have been due to genuine differences in rehabilitation potential.
Alternatively, given the limited employment of comprehensive
assessment by the community hospitals, it seems likely that other
factors influenced the predischarge planning process. There is, for
example, some indication that age itself was a factor in the referral
process, with discharge planners and physicians more interested in
the rehabilitation of younger patients or less confident in the ability
of older patients to benefit from continued rehabilitation. Older
stroke patients were, for example, more likely to be discharged to
long-term care facilities than to rehabilitation hospitals. Older hip
fracture patients were the most likely to be returned home with
limited nursing services.

There is also a question regarding the extent to which the patient's individual rehabilitation needs entered into the selection of
providers for continuing care. In the case of extended care facilities,
the patients mentioned physician preference, geographic location,
cost, and bed availability as the major considerations underlying

selection. In the cases of community-based programs, almost universal referral to the community's Visiting Nurse Association—to the exclusion of alternative rehabilitation providers—suggests a more routinized than individualized discharge planning process.

Finally, the comments of both patients and discharge planners suggest that nonreferral at discharge may, in many instances, have been the product of poor coordination rather than the absence of need:

> Nobody told us anything about what to do when I got home. We went to our summer cottage since everything is on one floor. My husband went to the high school to find a girl to help out while he was at work.

> *(Patient recollection)*

> Generally things go smoothly. Sometimes, though, the patient's physician will visit in the morning and tell them "you're going home today." By the time I find out about it they're gone.

> *(City Hospital Discharge Planner)*

Extending the Rehabilitation Process

As might be expected, the management of those patients transferred to the region's rehabilitation hospitals more closely approximated the philosophy of comprehensive rehabilitation. Typically, an extensive evaluation at admission was followed by an aggressive approach to the rehabilitation process. Almost all of the patients and their families remarked on the contrasting approaches of the community and rehabilitation hospitals:

> I wasn't doing so good at the hospital, so they sent me to the rehabilitation hospital. I got much better care there. I started to get physical therapy again. They didn't just let me sit around. They made me get up and do things. My aunt was very surprised when she came to visit the first time and found out I could walk.

> *(Patient recollection)*

> The doctor at the rehabilitation hospital took me off those pills. She said they were the cause of my being so tired—because they were too strong.

> *(Patient recollection)*

The most striking contrast between the community hospital and the rehabilitation hospital was, however, the scope of the rehabilitation hospital's efforts. The intensive physical therapy received by the patients was normally complemented by occupational and (where necessary) speech therapy sessions. Individually tailored assistive devices were readily employed when needed. Moreover, all therapeutic approaches seemed to be oriented to regaining, not just ambulation skills, but the whole range of basic functional skills required for independence:

> They put him on a walker and taught him to walk up and down stairs. They taught him to feed himself with his left hand and to shave, too. He learned to dress himself with his left hand. He could barely walk when he went in. When he came out he was walking pretty good.

> *(Daughter's recollection)*

A good indication of the scope of the rehabilitation hospital's concern was the attention devoted to the patient's transition back to the community:

> I was afraid of cars and being around traffic, so the therapist would take me on the bus and then make me cross the street. This way I lost my fear of being out on my own.

> *(Patient recollection)*

> Before I left the hospital one of the therapists came to the house with me to make sure I could manage at home. She installed a special toilet seat, and gadgets so I could reach the kitchen cabinets and do the housework with one hand.

> *(Patient recollection)*

This attention to detail was likely to include a discharge referral to a rehabilitation program for continued therapy on an outpatient basis.

The rehabilitation experiences of those patients transferred directly to a long-term care facility were generally less satisfactory. While a number of LTC facilities in the region were known for their aggressive rehabilitation programs, getting to such a facility was largely a "hit or miss" proposition. In most instances, the patients received a limited course of physical therapy. In many instances they received less:

She was in the hospital three weeks, and then in the nursing home. They didn't take good care of her there. The nurses didn't seem to care. They didn't have compassion. I thought she would die if she stayed there so I stopped work and took care of her at home.

(Husband's recollection)

When I got out of the hospital I went to a convalescent home for seven weeks. They gave me a room and that's it. There was no therapy.

(Patient recollection)

Fortunately for such patients, their stay in a long-term care facility rarely precluded a more aggressive and comprehensive rehabilitation effort in the future. Virtually all of those transferred to LTC facilities were referred for outpatient services at discharge, typically to the Visiting Nurse Association. While these referrals may have been made primarily in the interests of securing home-based nursing care, they opened the door to reconsideration of the patient's rehabilitation potential by the rehabilitation-oriented visiting nurses.

Whether patients returned to the community directly from the community hospital or by way of an institutional setting, the Visiting Nurse Association was likely to play an important role if community-based services were employed at all. In the absence of a discharge or physician referral, the VNA was the most visible and accessible program for patients seeking assistance.

The VNA took an aggressive and comprehensive approach to rehabilitation. Based on an initial home assessment, the agency provided or contracted for needed nursing, supportive, and rehabilitation services whenever such services were reimbursable (and, sometimes, when they were not). In its coordinating role, the agency—like the rehabilitation hospital—paid particular attention to practical details which might make the difference between a successful and an unsuccessful rehabilitation effort. In addition to its employment of physical, occupational, and speech therapists, the agency evaluated and frequently modified the home environment to facilitate patient independence. The patient's nutritional status was monitored and Meals-On-Wheels services employed when required. The agency arranged transportation to physician appointments, and involved, counseled, and supported family members:

When I got home I could barely get out of bed. The visiting nurse came regularly and arranged for the therapists. They had me walking and doing exercises. It was the visiting nurses and therapists who were responsible for getting me back on my feet.

(Patient recollection)

I don't know what I would have done without them. Mother could get around with a walker, but needed help with everything else. The nurses came a couple of times a week, and then once a week. They would leave instructions for the home health aides.

(Daughter's recollection)

Although reimbursement criteria and professional norms limited the agency's ability to initiate such services on its own, the agency was willing to press the patients' physicians for the introduction of needed services when physician initiative was lacking. This aggressive stance was critically important in many cases. While both stroke and hip fracture patients reported frequent contact with their community physicians, the focus of this contact centered largely on traditional aspects of medical care. Over half of the stroke patients and two-thirds of the hip fracture patients indicated, for example, that their contacts with physicians were limited solely to "check-up and monitoring" functions.

While the Visiting Nurse Association's central role in the region's network of community-based rehabilitation services, its reliance on an initial assessment process, and its aggressive and comprehensive approach to rehabilitation helped to offset the routinized discharge referral practices of the community hospitals, community-based rehabilitation in the region was not without problems. As noted earlier, significant numbers of patients received no referrals for community-based services, or were referred to other providers who were less comprehensive in their orientation. Those patients whose physicians elected to utilize community hospital rehabilitation departments or proprietary agencies for therapy received, for example, a much narrower range of services. Moreover, physicians could, and occasionally did, override the service recommendations of the VNA:

The visting nurse recommended speech therapy after he got home. The doctor said "No," that it wasn't necessary.

(Wife's recollection)

The visiting nurse came two times to give me a bath and change the bed. The girl was very pleasant and efficient, but I didn't see her after that. She called the surgeon about therapy, but he said that I didn't need any.

(Patient recollection)

Even when referral to the VNA was timely, and the agency given a relatively free hand to initiate service, the rehabilitation process diverged from the ideals of comprehensive rehabilitation in a number of important ways. The failure of the agency and the community hospitals to work together in discharge planning before the patient was returned to the community jeopardized continuity of the patient care process. There was little evidence that the agency drew upon earlier evaluations by the hospital rehabilitation departments. While the VNA's approach to rehabilitation was comparatively comprehensive, referrals for psychological or social services were rare. The agency tended to focus on nursing and home care services which were directly under its control and clearly reimbursable as part of the patient's posthospital convalescence. The comments of patients and agency personnel suggest that the duration of services provided through the agency was often determined by reimbursement guidelines rather than individual patient needs:

It would be good to have the therapy occasionally because it helps me keep going. But I guess I've used up my benefits. After all of the doctor bills I don't have any money.

(Patient statement)

This is one area where we function differently from a lot of agencies. Once they get people to the point where they can maintain themselves they pretty much withdraw. We try to hold on a little longer, but it's not easy. The services just aren't covered if you can't show dramatic gains.

(VNA rehabilitation nurse)

Finally, while the VNA was a major source of referrals to agencies other than those with which it contracted for services, it was likely to delay referral until its own contact with the patient was terminated. This was particularly true of referrals to agencies such as the Outpatient Rehabilitation Center which might have challenged the VNA's role as coordinator of the rehabilitation process. In principle, the division of labor between the VNA and the Center—

with the former providing home care services and the latter providing outpatient services—should have allowed a smooth transition
from one agency to the other. Like the other rehabilitation providers
in the region, however, the Center required its own mandate for
involvement in the patient care process (in the form of physician
referral), conducted its own comprehensive assessment of patient
needs, and insisted on coordinating all health, rehabilitation, and
social services other than those provided by the patient's community
physicians. These policies, coupled with the VNA's tendency to delay
referral to the Center, resulted in weeks or months of inactivity for
the patient before the initiation of Center therapy. It is not surprising
that many of those patients in the study who were referred to the
Center, facing yet another comprehensive assessment and weeks of
waiting, simply withdrew from one of the most extensive outpatient
rehabilitation services in the region.

Ironically, it was the Outpatient Rehabilitation Center's executive director who most clearly summed up the problems of interor-
ganizational cooperation in community-based rehabilitation:

> The system? What system? This region is one of the richest areas with
> respect to rehabilitation resources that I have seen. But we are the worst
> with respect to "dis-coordination." I used to think that it was that we
> were just learning to work together. I do not think so now. Where we
> have done it, it has been forced upon us by governmental edict or by
> payment. It is almost never a gut reaction.

> *(Rehabilitation Center executive director)*

Implications for Geriatric Services

The New England health planning region described here contained a
wealth of institutional and community-based rehabilitation providers. Under the best of conditions this array of largely autonomous
providers functioned as a loosely coordinated services delivery network. Often, the organizational complexity of the rehabilitation arena precluded the achievement of even moderate levels of integration
and continuity in the delivery of rehabilitation services. Many providers maintained a commitment to the ideals of aggressive, comprehensive, and individualized rehabilitation. These commitments,
however, were tempered by the peculiarities of each provider's organizational setting. In the absence of collective responsibility for pa-

tient progress through the acute and postacute phases of rehabilitation, there were few incentives for provider cooperation in patient assessment, the setting of long-term rehabilitation goals, or the delivery of medical, rehabilitation, and social services. Reimbursement criteria conceptualizing the rehabilitation effort as part of a postacute hospital convalescence, establishing predetermined periods of therapy, and requiring the demonstration of dramatic improvements in patient functioning, further routinized the delivery of rehabilitation services.

While all of the patients in the study encountered these organizational problems, the geriatric patients—with their multiple pathologies and limited social and economic resources—were at a particular disadvantage. Their problems were compounded by health care providers who were less likely to see "rehabilitation potential" in an elderly patient. To the extent that the study focused on "successful cases" (patients who eventually returned to the community), it probably underestimates the extent of the barriers to comprehensive rehabilitation of the elderly.

The study's geriatric patient career data suggest that a number of prerequisites must be met if elderly patients are to receive and benefit from existing rehabilitation services when they are needed. Central among these prerequisites are: (1) a better understanding of geriatric rehabilitation potential among those community and hospital-based physicians who control the patient care process; (2) greater intra- and interinstitutional cooperation among medical, rehabilitation, and support services; (3) expansion of the rehabilitation capabilities of geriatric service providers, especially long-term care facilities; and (4) flexible third-party reimbursement criteria which can accommodate the modest but critical functional gains often associated with the rehabilitation of elderly patients.

As important, the service delivery patterns emerging from the study raise important issues about the overall development of geriatric health and social services. There are significant parallels between the historical development of rehabilitation services during the first half of this century and the current emergence of geriatric services. Geriatric services are developing in a highly charged social and political context. Those who support their development are prompted by a range of motives and hold diverse if not conflicting visions of the ultimate nature and shape of such services. While this broad-based support is probably necessary for the further development of geriatric services, there is a real possibility that the recent expansion of federal entitlement, reimbursement, demonstration, research, and training programs in the field of aging will lead to a similar organizational dilemma: that is, a complex network of special geriatric programs and personnel that will make the holistic philosophy underlying the geriatric services movement extremely difficult to put into practice.

If such hazards are to be minimized, it is important to seriously consider the extent to which we want to, must, or can operationalize a holistic model of geriatric care, and then to act accordingly at the organizational level.

It may be that we will be satisfied to broaden the scope and improve the technical quality of existing services for the elderly. In this case, it may be sufficient to push for the sponsorship and development of new kinds of programs which fill the current gaps, and to concentrate on training health professionals whose disciplinary skills are tailored to the special needs of elderly patients—institutional-based consultant geriatricians, geriatric nurse practitioners, geriatric physical therapists, and similar health professionals skilled in relating to and managing the diseases of old age. We are beginning to move in this direction and the result is likely to be more appropriate and effective care for those elderly who are referred to the new geriatric services and personnel.

Alternatively, we may seek to improve the accessibility as well as the availability of new and existing geriatric services. To the extent that limited access to geriatric services is a function of restrictive entitlement criteria, it may be enough to work towards a broadening of these criteria. To the extent, however, that it is a function of sheer organizational complexity, it may be necessary to supplement the training of new geriatric health professionals with a thorough grounding in the structure of health services and reimbursement criteria, and to prepare them for aggressive patient advocacy as well as patient care roles.

Unfortunately, the study of rehabilitation services reported here confirms the frequent observation that availability and accessibility of relevant health care services do not guarantee their utilization. It does, however, suggest possible avenues for improving the chances of appropriate utilization. Certainly, the key role played by the patient's community physician in the employment of rehabilitation services affirms the appropriateness of current efforts to expose all physicians-in-training to the unique health problems associated with aging and to the potential contributions of specially-trained geriatric health personnel and targeted geriatric services. Similarly, it may yet be possible to achieve systematic consideration of geriatric service alternatives by organized health care providers through a quasiregulatory process similar to the discharge plan requirement associated with Medicare reimbursement. In the community under study, this requirement did facilitate contact with community-based services despite the routinized nature of the discharge planning process.

In its fullest expression, implementation of a holistic approach to geriatric care would require more than the presence, accessibility, or even utilization of a collection of special services for the elderly. It would require a fundamental change in the *way* such services are delivered. As suggested earlier, this would mean the provision of such services based on individual patient needs, in an integrated fashion, over time. Based on the experiences of the study's elderly stroke and hip fracture patients, it seems unlikely that this kind of sophisticated care can be achieved as long as the component parts are housed in a variety of organizationally autonomous units and programs. Should we aspire to this level of geriatric care in the near future, we will have to begin—and soon—to think in terms of more complex multilevel geriatric service systems, to work towards their development, and to prepare geriatrically-oriented health professionals who are able and willing to work effectively in them.

Notes

[1]Richard A. Lusky, "Ideological and Interest Group Barriers to Comprehensive Rehabilitation of the Physically Disabled." (Doctoral Dissertation, University of Connecticut, 1980).
[2]Glen Gullickson, & Sidney Licht, "Definition and Philosophy of Rehabilitation Medicine," in Sidney Licht (ed.), *Rehabilitation and Medicine* (Baltimore: Waverly Press, 1968), pp. 4–7.
[3]Albert F. Wessen, "The Rehabilitation Apparatus and Organization Theory," in Marvin B. Sussman (ed.), *Sociology and Rehabilitation* (Washington, D.C.: American Sociological Association, 1965), p. 162.
[4]Robert Straus, *Medical Care for Seaman: The Origin of Public Medical Services in the United States* (New Haven: Yale University Press, 1950); and Robert Straus, "Social Changes and the Rehabilitation Concept," in Sussman, *Sociology and Rehabilitation,* pp. 1–34.
[5]Marvin B. Sussman, "The Disabled and the Rehabilitation System," in Gary L. Albrecht (ed.), *The Sociology of Physical Disability and Rehabilitation* (Pittsburgh: University of Pittsburgh Press, 1972), pp. 223–256.
[6]Straus, "Social Change and the Rehabilitation Concept," pp. 111–112.
[7]Charles D. Bonner, *Medical Care and Rehabilitation of the Aged and Chronically Ill,* 3rd ed. (Boston: Little Brown and Co., 1974), p. 146.
[8]Wessen, "Rehabilitation Apparatus," p. 155.

[9]Rosemary Stevens, *American Medicine and the Public Interest* (New Haven: Yale University Press, 1971), pp. 328–330.

[10]For details on the rise of these rehabilitation-related occupations, see Eliot A. Krause, "Structured Strain in a Marginal Profession: Rehabilitation Counseling," *Journal of Health and Human Behavior* 6:1 (1965); Ruben J. Margolin, & Alan B. Sostek, "Professional Development and Training in Rehabilitation Administration and Supervision," *Journal of Rehabilitation* 34:3 (1968), pp. 18–20; and Richard T. Smith, "Health and Rehabilitation Manpower Strategy: New Careers and the Role of the Indigenous Paraprofessional," *Social Science and Medicine* 7 (1973): 281–290.

[11]For a review of the use of the patient career model in a study of chronic disease management, see Sidney H. Croog, S. Levine, and Z. Lurie, "The Heart Patient and the Recovery Process," *Social Science and Medicine* 2 (1968): 111–164.

[12]The tracer disease technique has most frequently been utilized in assessing the quality of medical care rendered by a single organized health care provider. See David M. Kessner, C. Kalk, and J. Singer, "Assessing Health Quality: The Case for Tracers," *New England Journal of Medicine* 268:4 (1973), pp. 189–194; Stephen R. Smith, "Application of the Tracer Technique in Studying Quality of Care," *Journal of Family Practice,* 1: 3–4 (1974), pp. 38–42.

[13]Joint Committee for Stroke Facilities, "Stroke Rehabilitation," *Stroke 3,* (1972), p. 360.

[14]S. C. Gallannaugh, "Regional Survey of Femoral Neck Fracture," *British Medical Journal* 2 (1976):1496.

[15]T. Glyn Thomas, & R. S. Stevens, "Social Effects of Fracture of the Neck of the Femur," *British Medical Journal* 3 (1974): 458.

[16]Figures on survivorship in stroke from Harry T. Zankel, *Stroke Rehabilitation* (Springfield: Charles C. Thomas, 1971), p. 5; Figures on survivorship in hip fracture from Thomas and Stevens, "Social Effects of Fracture," p. 456.

[17]Lionel B. Truscott, "Early Rehabilitative Care in Community Hospitals: Effect of Quality of Survivorship Following Stroke," *Stroke* 5 (1974): 623–629.

[18]C. M. Wylie, "Cues to Stroke Rehabilitation Referral Among Family Physicians," *Journal of American Geriatrics Society* 17 (1969):549–554; J. T. Lehman, B. J. DeLateur, R. S. Fowler, C. Warren, R. Arnhold, G. Schertzer, R. Hurka, J. Whitmore, A. Masock, and K. Chambers, "Stroke: Does Rehabilitation Affect Outcome?" *Archives of Physical Medicine and Rehabilitation* 56 (1975): 375–382.

[19]D. S. Muckle, "Fractures of the Femoral Neck, Parts I and II," in D. S. Muckle (ed.), *Femoral Neck Joint Fractures and Hip Joint Fractures* (New York: John Wiley & Sons, 1977).

[20]Thomas and Stevens, "Social Effects of Fracture."

[21]Rodney K. Beals, "Survival Following Hip Fracture," *Journal of Chronic Diseases* 22 (1972):235–244.

15

A Program for Preventive and Supportive Care of the Troubled Elderly

MILDRED ZIMMERMAN AND PHYLLIS KULTGEN

Introduction

The growing field of psychogeriatric medicine attests to an expanding recognition of the biomedical and psychosocial overlap which often occurs when comprehensive treatment of the troubled elderly is undertaken. It is our contention here, however, that recognition of the overlap is skewed in the direction of severe pathology. This probable imbalance may not be recognized by clinicians who practice in settings serving only the most severely disabled and disturbed but it is immediately evident to those who concentrate on the psychosocial side of the scale. It is important to redress the imbalance, we believe, so that a wide array of supportive social interventions may be provided to those under stress and those experiencing temporary deviations from the normal. The tasks of this chapter are to: (1) refine the interplay of medical, psychiatric, and social interventions by making distinctions which facilitate the task of outlining a program for preventive and supportive care, (2) identify general social services as distinct from what we call supportive social interventions, and (3) propose a program of support utilizing social interventions.

Distinctions

As our main concern is support for positive mental health, we begin by pointing to the confusion in the "aging" literature regarding referents for the terms "mental health", "mental illness", and "mental disease". Although "mental disease" seems restricted (for the most part) to disease states falling under the heading of "dementia" the reference is not always clear. But confusion here is minimal when it is compared to the unrestrained chaos surrounding the usage of the terms "mental health" and "mental illness". Sometimes these terms are used to refer to opposite poles of an implied continuum and at other times they are used interchangeably as a device to avoid repetitious phrasing. An extreme example of the confusion that engulfs the concepts appears in articles discussing varieties of mental illness followed by suggestions for mental health treatment.

Some of the confusion surrounding the two terms "mental illness" and "mental health" might be resolved by thinking of the concepts as categories rather than as two ends of a continuum. And at the same time, it would give each concept more explanatory power. That is, if mental health is a concept qualitatively distinct from mental illness one can seek ways of preserving some degree of mental health even though an individual is faced with some degree of mental illness (functional) or mental disease (organic). Using Jahoda's (1958) definition of mental health, that is, some degree of positive self attitudes, growth and self-actualization, integration of personality, autonomy, reality perception and self mastery, it can be asserted that some, if not all, of those dimensions of health can conceivably be maintained in the face of mental disease and mental illness. As a case in point, "an individual may suffer progressive organic brain deterioration and yet, within the limits of decreasing self-awareness and ability, be able to maximize the effectiveness of his behavior. . . . Presumably the more mentally healthy individual, with a late-life organic mental illness, will maintain the emotional, social, and physical demands of the environment at a more tolerable level than would be the case of the less mentally healthy individual."[1]

Mental illness is a category for which we have no well-conceived referents. Consider depression, reportedly the most common disorder in late life. We do not deny the existence of depressive disorders of a severe and recurrent nature such as bipolar illnesses and conditions diagnosed as "melancholia."[2] The pathology in these cases usually has a history, and in some cases—such as the manic-depressive, for example—a chemical or organic problem exists (or is at least assumed to be present). "Clinical depression" is further defined by the presence of sleep and/or appetite disturbances, difficulty concentrating, loss of interest in normal activities, bodily symptoms that have no physical basis, and so on. From 30 to 50 percent of the elderly in psychiatric ambulatory care settings suffer from clinical depression according to recent estimates.[3]

The point is that when severe depressive disorders are found in the elderly, they have been presumed to be untreatable which, in our terms, translates into the denial of the possibility of a positive mental health status for victims of severe depressive disorders. But recently, many clinicians have found that older adults are as responsive to counseling and psychotherapy as their younger counterparts. Also, much of the depression in the older population is now viewed as a product of the stresses of aging and, in many cases, is amenable to intervention and/or prevention. Although the symptoms may be rather severe, they can be alleviated and normal mood level restored with proper medication and therapy. We would like, therefore, to consider some of these types of clinical depression as deviations from a positive mental health status rather than definitive examples of mental illness.

Within this same context, we observe that many of those who work with the elderly see enough depression to believe that most everyone will experience at least *some* level of depressive symptoms at *some* point during his later life. With the multiplicity of losses and change, a milder form of depression becomes manifest as the elderly resign themselves to a negative view of aging and/or accept a life style that offers little stimulation or involvement in the world around them.

Unless the symptoms persist or become inordinately severe, however, "milder" forms of depression are not viewed as a clinical problem in the traditional medical and psychiatric sense of the word. In fact, some authorities have gone so far as to suggest that "normal aging" with its losses and change involves a number of such reactions that are not "true depression."[4] Similarly, Zung[5] has attempted to establish a baseline of depressive symptoms in the "normal elderly." We do not concur that depression is a normal part of aging any more than it is a normal part of adolescence or midlife, although the problem is a common one at all stages of life. Rather, we assert that depression is a major problem threatening mental health in late life.

Although it has been suggested that thinking of mental health as a category can, under some circumstances, be advantageous, the issue of category versus continuum is not one of major importance.

However, establishing clear referents for the term "mental health" is important. At the least it is *not* mental illness and because it is not, we urge others to drop the phrase "mental health problem" from usage. As indicated earlier, mental health refers here to positive self-attitudes, integration of personality, growth, autonomy, and so forth. Presumably all of these can be operationalized.[6] Difficulties of measurement aside, the claim is made that referents for these components of health can be identified. But if this is the case, what in addition to Jahoda's list of positive attributes does the term "mental health" connote? For this purposes of the discussion, the term "mental health" refers to services which both enhance health and prevent the loss of health. Such services include what are often referred to as general social services and services we choose to characterize as supportive social interventions. We concentrate on the latter category of service because it is here that the opportunities for intervention offer hope for successful restoration to a positive mental health status for persons "at risk" of deviations from the normal. Prior to the discussion of supportive social interventions, the distinction between these and general social services is outlined.

In a sense, the wide net of general social services provided by a government (and which undergird a society) are mental health services. Hedges against unemployment, educational opportunities, public physical health programs including nutrition programs, housing programs—any service which attempts to improve the quality of life for the governed—should promote mental health. But this aspect of general public health is based on an assumption not always clarified. Made explicit that assumption reads: When a society is healthy its members have an opportunity to be healthy. This is one basis for adherence to social psychiatry, that is, a positive social environment promotes healthy individuals.

Having acknowledged the importance of general services, we move on to an identification of more directly supportive interventions.

Supportive Social Intervention

The underlying assumption here reflects the very basic psychosociological insight that an individual's identity and self-concept are shaped within group contexts. That is, individual identity is largely formed by "hooking in" to existing social structures. Paradoxically then, autonomy, self-mastery, and self-actualization are nourished within supportive social networks. The tension existing between the tyranny of group pressures and individual development is one, we assert, that has been resolved by mentally healthy aging individuals. Yet the person who has depended on group-oriented options for successful development may find these drastically reduced in later years.

Important social group contacts for the aging person include family networks, informal peer groups, neighborhood networks, and, in many cases, a religious group network. Such a list suggests the existence of natural supporting networks. But when social statistics are reviewed one wonders how effective such networks are. Gene Cohen has made such a review under the heading of "social issues":

1. Isolation without adequate social supports is a critical issue. One in 7 men over age 65 lives alone. Nearly one-third of women 65 and older live by themselves.
2. Related to isolation is the loss of significant others. Seventeen percent of men 65 and older are widowed; 30 percent in the over-75 age group. With women, 54 percent age 65 and older are widowed; a startling 70 percent of the over-75 age group have lost their spouses.
3. The opportunity for man-woman relationships diminishes with age due to differential mortality rates. At age 65 there are 4 women to every 3 men; by age 85 women outnumber men 2 to 1 (US Dept. HEW, 1978).

Among Cohen's summary remarks he states: The dramatic growth of the older population (from 3 million [4 percent of the population] in 1900 to 22 million [10 percent of the population] in 1975) has been met by a societal failure to adequately meet either the individual or the group needs of the elderly. While programs like Social Security and Medicare attempt to respond to specific needs of the individual, comparable programs addressing such group needs as meaningful social and interpersonal involvements lag far behind. The mental health significance is obvious.[7] It is this lag to which supportive social interventions are addressed. Where natural supportive networks fail or become nonexistent, mental health is difficult to maintain; therefore, supportive social interventions may be considered primary prevention mechanisms when the individual is "at risk" because of societal or environmental failure. And in a secondary sense, supportive services are preventive: When an individual has slipped into the ill category, early intervention is called for. Counsel-

ing programs, including peer counseling, aimed at improving interactive skills, pastoral and medical counseling (and any other programs where the elderly receive advice form trusted confidants) come
under the heading of supportive social interventions. Such intervention services are underdeveloped and among those that should concern mental health personnel. Consequently, it is our intention to
suggest a program that proposes intervention strategies for use by
specific professionals and paraprofessional counselors serving the
elderly.

A Proposed Model of Support

With the number of older people increasing, attention to the many
changes they go through suggests a monumental need, one that goes
far beyond the capacities of any one profession or even a group of
professions. One focus of mental health and the elderly obviously lies
in the area of education and the correction of stereotypes and misinformation. A second focus is that of supporting individuals as they
learn to cope and make maximal adaptations. Concentrating on these
two areas we would like to suggest the importance of the development of psychosocial support at a number of different points in the
elderly person's social environment. If we cannot reshape our whole
society to make it a more favorable place to live out one's later years,
we can at least establish a system of supports that are accessible and
acceptable to the older adult. Several possible categories of support
figures are likely. We would like to limit this discussion to the
following six such prospects: the elderly themselves as a group,
health professionals, specific members of the elderly's peer group, the
family, the clergy, and those in the network of services and organizations that have regular contact—senior center staff, meal site personnel, home health aides, and other related agency workers. The function and role of each of these supporters/counselors will be described,
and a model of preventive mental health care will be proposed.

The Supporters/Counselors and Their Roles

The Elderly as a Group. First and foremost, the elderly themselves
should have broad exposure to the model. They may not necessarily
be interested in becoming counselors themselves, but would benefit
from the educational emphasis. After all, the elderly share with
others the same misinformation about aging. They could also help to

diffuse or disperse the intentions of the program. Their role in the program should be obvious. They are the target group, and it is most important to begin with a broad general campaign for implementation of the program that includes as many of the elderly as possible.

The Health Professional as Counselor. The elderly tend to place a great deal of confidence in the health team. The nurse and physician are trusted figures, and medical authority and knowledge command utmost respect. This deference puts the health team in a position of major influence and offers them the opportunity for an unlimited positive (or negative) impact.

Witness the degree to which the elderly confide in their physician or nurse. A study of family physicians in Missouri revealed that depression and isolation (living alone) were two of the five most common presenting problems of older patients. A surprising 80 percent of the physicians stated that their older patients came to them with sexual problems; and nearly half (49.7 percent) of the respondents reported that they had had an older patient who had committed suicide.[8] Pressure on the health team to address mental health issues as well as biomedical concerns seems to be mounting. The President's Commission on Mental Health urged collaboration of health and mental health and, in 1979, the National Institute of Mental Health held an invitational conference, "Mental Health Services in Primary Care Settings."[9] The summary of the conference (HEW, 1979) mentioned no specific age group, but cited the need to correlate the physical problems more systematically with behavioral or emotional problems in screening, evaluation, and treatment. Psychiatrists have also urged primary care physicians to be alert to mental health issues with elderly patients and their families, and to be prepared to intervene.[10] Still others who have studied the high rate of suicide among elderly males have argued for more education for physicians in these critical matters. According to these investigators, about three-quarters of the elderly who take their own lives see a physician within a month before their deaths.[11]

Additional demands on the health care professions to provide supportive care to those at risk of losing a positive mental health status must seem overwhelming at times. The model elaborated below will provide some organization and limits—at least for preventive care.

The Elderly's Peers as Counselors. A number of highly successful programs have developed across the country for training elderly "natural helpers" to work as "peer counselors." These paraprofession-

als are usually selected for their warmth and empathy and they have
the respect of their peers. They are given extensive training and
supervision, and, although programs vary, the main idea and
claimed secret to success is that the elderly see a peer as a valuable
counselor because very simply the peer has "been there." Just as
many alcoholics feel that other alcoholics are their best source of
help, so also do many elderly feel their experience is unique to their
age group. For a number of other reasons, a peer counselor seems to
work well with the elderly.

Some of those who have benefited from their association with a
peer counselor insist that the person comes to fill the void left by the
death of a spouse or close family member. A trainer of peer counselors
has noted that peers are less likely to invoke dependence on the part
of the counselee than is a younger service worker. Perhaps most
important, Waters points out, the peer counselor serves as a role
model for the older client. With a role model, the elderly counselee
can see ways to cope with problems and to react to life as an aging
individual.[12]

The enthusiasm of participants, recipients, and directors of these
programs is impressive. The peer counselors themselves appear to
benefit immeasurably from their involvement. They experience
growth in their self-awareness and coping abilities, and many find
that the group of peer counselors provides its members important
support as they continue to meet for supervision or to discuss their
own problems. As counselors to other elderly, the peers feel needed
and they view themselves as performing a valuable service. Overall,
the peer counselor occupies a much different role in the life of the
elderly individual than does the health professional.

The Family as Counselors. The family has been shown to persist in
maintaining ties with aging parents and relatives. Contacts are
frequent[13] and the modified-extended family continues to exist
throughout the life course.[14] Nonetheless, families often feel totally
confused and unclear on how to respond to an aging parent or relative
and find they need assistance from professionals.

The stress on the family who is caring for a disabled elderly
relative is enormous, and marked changes in a family's relationships
can result when a relative enters the home. Kirschner suggests an
ecological perspective for helping families; that is, the full environment is considered rather than just individual personalities or
problems.[15] As part of the ecological view, a family would have access
to a variety of professionals and community resources, thereby deriv-

ing some relief from sharing its responsibility. At least family members would not feel all alone with the problem. Others have found that support groups for families give effective mutual support.

The family is an important source of morale for the elderly. Many elderly are hesitant to depend on their children, but during a crisis the family of necessity becomes especially important. As counselors who provide ongoing support and acceptance, the family is invaluable. Those elderly who are without family ties are indeed unfortunate. A substitute family may be needed to close this gap.

The Clergy as Counselors. The elderly often place as much confidence in their clergy as they do in their physicians. Religious ties are a primary source of support and comfort, and can be a powerful influence in the promotion of mental health. Many clergy act as counselors, but whether or not they engage heavily in "pastoral care," they are privy to the personal lives of many of their congregations. Those clergy who see themselves as counselors should be included in our proposed counselor network, and it is, therefore, equally important for all clergy to have accurate information about aging because they have an important educational function within their congregations as well as within the community.

Personnel in the Aging Network as Counselors. The "aging network" is a term often used by elderly service workers to refer collectively to the full range of services provided through the Older Americans Act, retiree organizations, and individuals or agencies that share an interest in the well-being of older adults. Counseling has not, for the most part, been a part of the aging network; and community mental health services have not, in most places, become integrated into the network. The barriers to providing mental health or counseling services to the elderly are becoming more understood.[16] The elderly apparently see mental health as a threat, or they simply do not appreciate its conception and function. Viewing the problem from the community mental health standpoint, few mental health professionals are trained to work with the older adult, and administrators have been reluctant to foster services. A joint project by the American Personnel and Guidance Association and the Administration on Aging has attempted to break through these barriers and train more people to do gerontological counseling. Also, some regional Area Agencies on Aging are laying plans to develop comprehensive care umbrellas for the elderly that include counseling and mental health. These and other measures may help narrow the gap.

Meanwhile, the service staff in the aging network are viable candidates to include in our counselor scheme. Typically, these workers are very dedicated to and concerned for the elderly. Furthermore, they are the "front line," the ones with regular, even daily contact with their clients. A case can be made for citing this group of paraprofessionals as the ones with the most potential influence. They not only have the most frequent contact, they also are usually indigenous to the area and know best how to communicate with the elderly. Common turf and common language are important allies, possibly the most valuable allies to have in home health care, daily hot lunch programs, and senior citizen centers.

Preventive/Supportive Mental Health Care for the Elderly

In order to fulfill their roles as formal or informal support persons for the aged, some guidelines need to be established for the five categories of counselors. A four-part plan is proposed as a program of information and skill from which the counselors may proceed: basic knowledge of aging, communication skills, the relevance of social support, and autonomy and dependence in late life. These four areas may constitute the training package for the counselors, and this content may also serve as a guide to interaction with the elderly.

Basic Knowledge of Aging

The counselors should be well-versed in accurate information about the aging process. They need to know what is normal and what is pathological; they should understand and be able to empathize with the elder's losses; they should be able to counter inaccurate or stereotypical views of aging; their attitudes should reflect a healthy and realistic approach towards aging in general and their own aging in particular. Memory and aging is perhaps one of the most misunderstood, misinterpreted concerns.

The multitude of research findings about memory and aging is becoming increasingly clear: the effect of growing older on our memory capacities is significant. Memory is strongly tied to the cognitive system.[17] Regularly, we use cues of various kinds to help us remember shopping needs, when certain events happened, and other associations that aid recall. Many memory problems, Kausler asserts, are attention problems or *in*attention problems; we simply do not focus on an event well enough to remember it. Even short-term memory, Kausler insists, is stable through the seventies. These important *facts* refute common misconceptions. Our counselors should be well-informed.

Communication Skills

Some primary concepts and skills in communication serve as useful helping tools and also define or restrict the counselor's role to that of supportive confidants. There is no need for the counselor to become a "therapist," and techniques more commonly used in psychotherapy require more training than is feasible in this context. Rather, the counselor is one who has well-developed listening skills and is able to respond appropriately and with awareness of his or her own feelings and thoughts. Communication skills often used in this framework are: listening skills, responding skills, and problem-solving skills.[18] A brief description of each of these follows:

Listening. A number of aids to developing helping skills have been designed in the past decade.[19] Carkhuff's "core conditions" of effective communication are: accurate empathy, warmth or respect, genuineness, concreteness, self-disclosure, immediacy, and confrontation. Listening and empathic responses are key elements, and techniques to increase these skills have proven to be successful. Carkhuff, for example, developed scales to assess listening and empathic understanding. A counselor can improve listening skills by classifying his or her response and locating it on the scale. Some listening and empathic skills are natural—at least some people seem to have a natural talent for them. Refined and well-developed listening skill is more rare and is difficult to achieve. Those who regularly work with these skills regularly believe that our daily communication is so limited that we rarely move beyond the exchange of information about problems or topics. Only when we reach the third level of Carkhuff's scale do we begin to hear and respond to the content of what is said *and* hear and respond to the feelings. And this is where the minimal facilitative function starts.

Responding. Guides for helpful responding usually start with the helper's self-awareness. In order to be empathic and "tune in" to another person, a helper must be clear about his or her own feelings and able to concentrate on the client. Each communicant is then a separate person. Projections and assumptions are minimized and the exchange presents a greater opportunity for clarity.

Skilled responding also involves knowing how to ask questions, knowing when to support a person and when to confront, making judgments about when and how to exert influence, and when to use self-disclosure. The following list of responses are known as "road-blocks to communication."[20] The roadblocks, initially devised for parent-child communication, have served as "golden rules" for many of those in the helping professions:

1. Ordering or commanding—can promote resistence or fear
2. Warning, threatening—can invite resentment or submissiveness
3. Moralizing, preaching—encourages guilt or defensiveness
4. Advising or sending solutions—causes dependency or resistence and implies the person cannot solve his or her own problem
5. Persuading with logic, arguing—promotes counterarguments and may cause the person to feel inferior
6. Judging, criticizing, blaming—implies incompetence, poor judgment
7. Praising, agreeing—implies high expectations, manipulation geared toward desired behavior
8. Name calling, ridiculing—invites low self-worth and feeling of being unlovable
9. Analyzing, diagnosing—threatening, the person may stop expression for fear of being exposed
10. Reassuring, sympathizing—the person may feel misunderstood
11. Probing, questioning—often is demanding and a distraction from the problem
12. Diverting, sarcasm, withdrawal—implies problem is unimportant, or that it should be avoided

It is important to remember that this list is applicable when the "helpee" is expressing a personal problem. In a medical setting, a health professional can hardly expect to stop "analyzing and diagnosing" or asking questions. However, such behavior is likely to block the disclosure of personal matters (as opposed to medical), if these more intimate issues are also analyzed and classified by the nurse or physician. Likewise, reassurance may stop communication; a person may be left thinking, "I guess I'm not supposed to feel this way." Many helpers who rely on the roadblocks (sometimes called "the dirty dozen") find the list easier to avoid than one would first think. That they have withstood over ten years of use in a rapidly growing field in which other helping devices have proliferated would seem to confirm their validity.

Problem Solving. Exploring alternatives is an important part of the communicating and helping process. Problem solving actually requires astute use of the first two skills—listening and responding. With problem solving, however, the goal involves decision making on the part of the client.

Social Support and Health

The third component of the preventive model concerns the relevance of social support to the elderly. A body of recent research points to a link between social support and adaptation to stress. The important study of Berkman and Syme[21] gave the most conclusive evidence of the relationship between social support and mortality. Those in their study who had the fewest supports had a mortality rate more than twice as high as those having the greatest number of social bonds (such as marital ties, membership in organizations, etc.). Blazer found social support to be a significant empirical factor for the elderly.[22] Still others have suggested that a lack of social ties may be associated with ill health regardless of any pronounced stress factors.[23] The precise mechanism that makes social support so potent is not yet defined, but many now assert that it is critical because the relationship is so strong.

Weiss proposed six "provisions" which are supplied through social support: attachment, social integration, reassurance of worth, opportunity for nurturing others, reliable alliance, and obtaining help and guidance. Although these items cannot be declared as *the* final and vital components of a functional support system, they appear to be good working definitions for our counselors. Expanding on these characteristics slightly, and relating them to elderly individuals, their pertinence becomes obvious:

1. Attachments—long-term relationships, things having historical significance to the individual
2. Social integration—membership and belonging in social systems of meaning
3. Reassurance of worth—feedback that continues to reinforce self-esteem
4. Opportunity for nurturing others—opportunities to give in purposeful ways

5. Reliable alliance—social ties that can be depended upon
6. Obtaining help and guidance—being able to avail oneself of assistance when it is needed[24]

The counselors themselves may fulfill the need for attachment, reassurance of self-worth, and opportunity for nurturing others in the reciprocity of their relationship with the older individual. They may also become a reliable ally and facilitate the individual's need for help and guidance from other sources. The counselors also can assess their "clients'" social support as to its adequacy by using Weiss' components as an inventory check list. This critical area can be attended to specifically, and needed support incorporated or constructed when necessary.

Autonomy and Dependence in Late Life

Autonomy is an elusive term to define and it tends to have different meanings for different people. Generally, an autonomous person is one who behaves independently and makes selective choices even under considerable duress. A kind of creative self-direction is implied as well as a sense of mastery and self-control. The psychoanalytic school views "the self" (some use the term "inner self") to refer to the deeper identity of an individual, an identity other than the multiple roles and the outer manifestations of ego. Still others view autonomy as an internal anchoring of self-worth, a self-esteem that relies on an inner sense of value rather than on external love objects, roles, or accomplishments.

This discussion of the importance of autonomy should not be taken as reinforcement for the American credo of "rugged individualism." This credo has been held to be at least partly responsible for our "pursuit of loneliness" (Phillip Slater) and for our willingness to pretend that we should be self-reliant in all ways. Our critical need for social support was just mentioned along with empirical evidence indicating that human contact is apparently basic to our nature and our survival. As mentioned earlier, such dependence is not contradictory to the principle of autonomy. Rather, a strong sense of autonomy usually is perceived as an enabling factor for satisfying relationships. True autonomy acknowledges need, and leads to greater receptivity and increased interaction with others—including the need for more dependence as physical changes progress. Very plainly, autonomy is not to be confused with a turning inward, self-centeredness, isolation, or loss of interest in others. To the contrary, the development of underlying personal autonomy is a growth process.

The use of life review as a therapeutic tool with older adults has gained popularity recently and has been seen as an enhancement to autonomy. Life review and autonomy also fit in with the developmental psychologists' concepts of late life as a time of seeking completion and integration, active interior process, and acceptance of one's life as it has been.[25] Cohler reminds us that a number of studies have shown that continued family responsibilities for older women are associated with their low morale, and that many elderly prefer "intimacy at a distance" in family relationships.[26] Cohler theorizes that this preference for distance signifies the desire for inner reflection; he cites India and Japan as countries which provide "culturally determined solutions" to assist older family members' need for increased autonomy. In Hindi philosophy, for example, late life is the time for integrating oneself into the "cycle of lives" and for achieving inner calm, rather than for continuing to pursue filial obligations.

Regrettably, American culture does not provide such a framework. Perhaps, then, it falls on the care providers of the elderly to find ways other than life review alone to uphold the aging individual's sense of autonomy. If those who surround the disabled elderly build an "ecology of dependence" (Ian Lawson), they would do well also to foster an inner autonomy—the other side of the coin. Overhelping or "learned helplessness" would thereby have little chance of flourishing. Becoming more inner-directed and sharing the wisdom with others—including the care providers—would seem to invoke a mustering of resources and provide a sense of purpose.

The poem below expresses the idea most eloquently. It was written when the author was 80 years of age:

A Manifesto[27]

Come hell or high water
To hang on to the basics of being human

1.
Shrink as the world will
With all the disconnecting going on
Still to be a worlding self
Collect events and persons
that I care about
have enterprises in motion
even tho small
with many things to talk about.

2.

With life crowded with more and more
  frustrations
  defeats
  decline
    Still—
        a feeling for the God whom to serve is perfect freedom.

3.

With less body and mind
  to be sensitive with
With attention more clamored
  by my own needs and hurts

      Still to make persons present to me
      And understand their struggle to found a home place
        in a precarious world.

4.

Not to care about what happens
  is to be extinguished
    So even though it hurts
      and adds haunting burdens
        still to feelingly think

5.

Despite failing nerve synapses
And cortex power to mobilize all the consciousness I once was

  I shall continue to
  Turn lived moments into meanings which are me

  Continue
    to believe in certain possibilities

6.

Still to be an inner-personal region
  that has an identity
  makes choices
  interiorizes significant others
    I shall listen
    To what the highest and best said in their own heart
      as they fought their way thru

I shall yet
  be putting together an ecology of spirit

    that nourishes me.
    and to which I contribute.

7.

I am awesome Mystery
    which I will not profane or trivialize

Nor is anyone else
    to profane or trivialize.

8.

Still to be Spirit!
    though sometimes dim and murky

Still to be moments
    which light up with significances!

Even tho I am in process of disappearing
    Still to have a meaningful story
        since soon that will be all.

Ross Snyder

Conclusion

The plan presented here may seem ambitious and overly idealistic. Let us consider some possible objections:

The plan appears to be difficult to manage and coordinate and would demand full time attention from at least one person to administer. As presented above, such a program would indeed require a great deal of energy and ability to conduct and maintain. Further, the guarantee of a professional backup person for care consultation would be needed to assist those who need help with special clients. Supervision and continuing training would be needed, and new counselors would need to be trained, periodically.

Groups would not have to be trained in segregated fashion (as they have been listed and described above), however, and the network of trained counselors would be available to assist new trainees. The extent to which other elderly serving agencies would be involved, as well as a community-wide selection of clergy and families would further the coordination of services for the elderly and improve service delivery. The mere fact that there is a broad network of people sharing a common goal of improved contact with the elderly would result in more communication.

It is well established at this point that community mental health centers do not reach the elderly by waiting for them to enter the doors of clinics to become clients. Rather, the mental health professionals who work with the elderly must develop opportunities in the community and work to integrate mental health services with other programs for the elderly. In conducting the program described here, clinic personnel would have extensive contact in the community as leaders and as learners, and would be activating the community mental health concept through fostering the mutual-help philosophy.

So many people would need to be trained. Physicians would be reluctant to take the time for training or resist becoming part of the plan. Starting with a small pilot program, and then developing into a larger endeavor, would probably be advisable. Not every service worker, family member, clergy person, or physician would be effective as a counselor or would even want to try. The recruitment of counselors should be geared toward finding people with natural helping capacities: empathy, a desire to be helpful, and a genuine concern for the problem.

The inclusion of physicians would probably be difficult. Identification of a few physicians and other health providers who are interested would be instrumental. With their input, plans could be made for presenting the model through continuing education opportunities, local medical societies, and other available options.

Since the program is ambitious, its continuation into the future seems unlikely. Would not the long-term effect of such an effort be negligible? The success of the program would depend on the numbers of the people who eventually became involved, their enthusiasm and the overall effect of the program on the elderly themselves. The key factor is the outcome. If the older adults find the program beneficial and want it to continue, the broad network of helpers will remain on an ongoing basis.

Some counselors would be likely to drop out and others continue. The experience of most older adult peer counseling programs across the country is that turnover is small. Those who were trained in the initial stages have felt rewarded and have continued to be interested and active in their role.

With financial backing becoming increasingly difficult, the survival of such programs appears questionable. Cost effectiveness is an issue, and prevention programs are always subject to financial scrutiny because it is difficult to prove their value. We know immunization programs are valuable because of lowered prevalence and incidence of the diseases. Finding quantitative methods for measuring the impact of this program would be harder, but not impossible. To date, however, prevention programs for the elderly have not been developed to any degree, much less evaluated.

The costs for the program are less than might be at first assumed. Training costs would be a factor, and administration of the program would require a budget and at least one full-time director, depending on the size of the project. Some transportation costs would be necessary, mostly for the peer counselors who would otherwise not see their client (as would the family member, service worker from another agency, or clergy).

If community mental health centers were to be the organizers—and this seems logical although not necessarily the only way—budget considerations would undoubtedly be an issue. Some centers have conscientiously developed programs for the elderly and others have lagged behind. Apparently one of the main barriers to improved service delivery to the elderly lies not with the lack of counselor training nor with the lack of sophistication and willingness on the part of the elderly, but with the attitudes of the administrators of centers.[28] These attitudes are due to both the lack of priority for the mental health of the elderly, and a reluctance to invest in programs that are not income-producing.

Funding is undeniably a problem, but that does not mean that we need to abandon our vision of effective services. If enhancing the *quality* of life is as important as lengthening the *duration* of life, then we as professionals in "aging" must demand that a just share of societal resources be directed toward an improved social environment for our elders.

Notes

[1]James E. Birren, & Jayne Renner, "Concepts and Criteria of Mental Health and Aging," in J. E. Birren, and R. B. Sloan (eds.), *Handbook of Mental Health and Aging* (Englewood Cliffs, NJ: Prentice-Hall, 1980), pp. 4–33.

[2]APA, 1980.

[3]Daniel Blazer, *Depression in Late Life* (St. Louis: C. V. Mosby, 1982).

[4]Charles Gaitz, "Depression in the Elderly," in W. E. Fann, I. Karacan, A. D. Pokorny, and R. L. Williams et al. (eds.), *Phenomenology and Treatment of Depression* (Jamaica, New York: Spectrum Publications, 1977), pp. 153–166.

[5]William W. K. Zung, "Depression in the Normal Aged," *Psychomatics* 8:5 (1967), pp. 287–292.

[6]M. Jahoda, *Current Concepts of Positive Mental Health* (New York: Basic Books, 1958).

[7]G. Cohen, "Prospects for Mental Health and Aging," in J. E. Birren, and R. B. Sloan (eds.), *Handbook of Mental Health and Aging,* (Englewood Cliffs, NJ: Prentice-Hall, 1980).

[8]Kenneth Callen, S. Ingman & D. Lower, "Physicians' attitudes toward geriatric medical education." Unpublished manuscript, University of Missouri, Columbia, MO, (1980).

[9]U.S. Department of Health and Human Services. *Mental Health Services in Primary Care Settings,* Report of a conference, Washington, D.C., 1979.

[10]Daniel Blazer, & S. W. Friedman, "Depression in Late Life," *American Family Practitioner* 20:5 (November, 1979), pp. 91–96.

Kelly, John T., et al., "What the Family Physician Should Know About Treating Elderly Patients," *Geriatrics* 32:10 (October, 1977), pp. 79–92. Also see Bennet S. Gurian, "Psychogeriatrics and Family Medicine," *The Gerontologist* 15:4 (August, 1975), pp. 308–310.

[11]Marvin Miller, "Suicide After Sixty," *Aging* 289–290 (November-December, 1978), pp. 28–31.

Waters, Elinor, A. Weaver, & B. White, *Gerontological Counseling Skills: A Manual for Training Service Providers,* Continuum Center, Oakland University, Rochester, Michigan (1980).

[12]Elinor Waters, B. White, B. Dates, S. Reiter, & A. Weaver, *Peer Group Counseling for Older People: Final Report to the Administration on Aging,* Continuum Center, Oakland University, Rochester, Michigan (1980).

[13]Ethyl Shanas, "Social Myth as Hypothesis: The Case of the Family Relations of Old People," *The Gerontologist* 19 (1979): pp. 3–9.

[14]L. Ruben, *Worlds of Pain: Life in the Working Class Family* (New York: Basic Books, 1976).

G. Rosenbach, & D. Anspach, *Working Class Kinship* (Lexington, MA: D. C. Heath-Lexington Books, 1973).

[15]Charlotte Kirschner, "The Aging Family Crisis: A Problem in Living," *Social Casework* (April, 1979), pp. 209–216.

[16]Judith E. Hagebak, & B. R. Hagebak, "Serving the Mental Health Needs of the Elderly: The Case for Removing Barriers and Improving Service Integration," *Community Mental Health Journal* 16:4 (Winter, 1980), pp. 263–275; Birren and Renner, *Concepts and Criteria.*

[17]Donald Kausler, "Memory and Aging." Lecture for Multidisciplinary Seminars on Aging, University of Missouri, Columbia (March, 1981).

[18]Patricia Alpaugh, & M. Haney *Counseling the Older Adult,* (Los Angeles: University of Southern California Press, 1978).

[19]Gerard Egan, *The Skilled Helper* (Monterey, CA: Brooks/Cole, 1975).

Carkhuff, Robert, *Helping and Human Relations,* Vols. I and II. (New York: Holt, Rinehart and Winston, 1969).

[20]Thomas Gordon, *Parent Effectiveness Training* (New York: Peter Wyden, 1970).

[21]Lisa F. Berkman, & S. L. Syme, "Social Networks, Host Resistance and Morality: A Nine-year Followup Study of Alameda County Residents," *American Journal of Epidemiology* 109:2 (1979): 186–204.

[22]Daniel Blazer, "Social Support as a Predictor of Mortality in a Community Sample of Older Adults," *The Gerontologist* 20:5, Part II (November, 1980), p. 67.

[23]P. M. Marvin, & J. G. Ingham, "Friends, Confidants and Symptoms," *Social Psychiatry* 11 (1976): 51–58.

[24]R. S. Weiss, "The Provisions of Social Relationships," in Ruben, Z. (ed.), *Doing Unto Others* (Englewood Cliffs, NJ: Prentice-Hall, 1974).

[25]Bernice Neugarten, "Personality Change in Late Life: A Developmental Perspective," in Eisdorfer and Lawton (eds.), *The Psychology of Adult Development and Aging,* Washington. D. C., American Psychological Association, 1973, pp. 311–335.

Eriksen, Erik, *Childhood and Society* (New York: W. W. Norton, 1950).

Buhler, Charlotte, "The General Structure of the Human Life Cycle," in *The Course of Human Life,* C. Buhler and F. Massarik (eds.), New York: Springer, (1968).

[26]L. Rosemary, and E. Kockeis, "Predispositions for a Sociological Theory of Action and the Family," *International Social Science Journal* 15 (1963), pp. 410–426.

Cohler, Bertram J., "Autonomy and Interdependence in the Family of Adulthood," paper presented at 33rd Annual Meeting, Gerontological Society of America, San Diego, California (November, 1980).

[27]Ross Snyder, *A Manifesto* (unpublished poem).

[28]C. P. Pratt, & A. S. Kethley, "Anticipated and Actual Barriers to Developing Community Mental Health Programs for the Elderly," *Community Mental Health Journal,* Vol. 16, No. 3 (1980), pp. 205–216.

EPILOGUE:
A PERSONAL MEMOIR

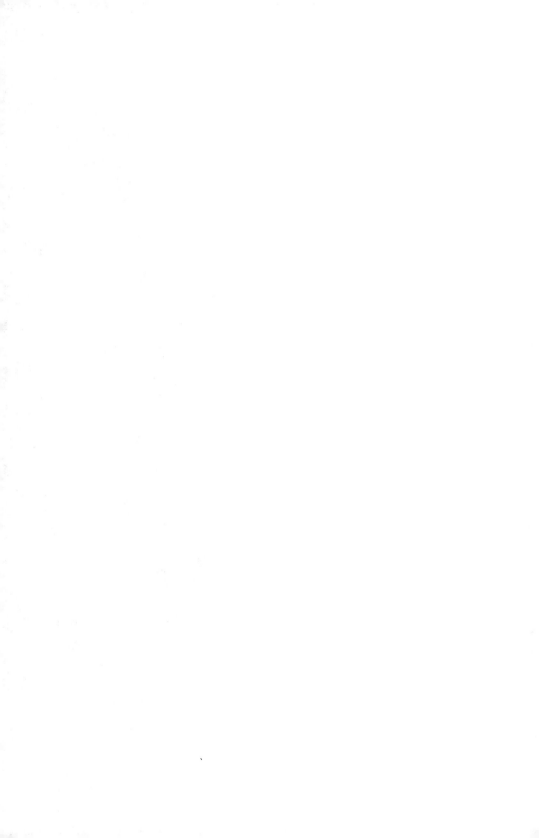

16

The Disengagement of an Aging Activist: The Making and Unmaking of a Gerontologist

DONALD O. COWGILL

I have recently been elevated to that exalted status of Professor Emeritus. Emeritus means that while your real income is cut in half your "psychic" income is doubled!

The title of this chapter may give the impression that I am somewhat ambivalent about retirement. That is true. Robert Havighurst finds two distinct patterns of retirement among academics. There are those who make an abrupt, radical change, abandoning academic pursuits and contacts, usually changing residence, and often converting an erstwhile hobby into a full-time activity, perhaps even a business. The other pattern is one of continuity, with the individual continuing research, writing, occasional lecturing and, God forbid, even serving on committees! Ironically, though I have been studying retirement for forty years and find myself becoming more and more favorable to it as my personal encounter with it approaches, I still have moments of doubt about the best way for me to tackle retirement.

I stumbled into the study of gerontology before it had a name. I wrote my dissertation on "trailerites"—people who lived in trailers back in the days when "mobile homes" were still mobile. After collecting a sample from coast to coast and after being an observer and participant for three years, I discovered that one-third of my subjects were elderly and retired. This early research may have influenced my later encounters with gerontology. Here I found older people doing what they wanted to do, when they wanted to do it. This segment of the population had not yet been identified as a problem or targeted as a market. They were normal, natural human beings (not subjects). They were enjoying life.

In 1946 I went to Wichita State on a joint appointment; the Community Planning Council downtown payed one-third of my salary. My work with the Council kept me in close touch with the life and problems of the community. The research that I directed on their behalf was largely of an applied nature. I tried, however, to keep it attuned at the same time to the theoretical developments in my academic field. Some of the research and planning focused on the problems of older people in the community and thus I was led into further encounters with the field of gerontology. Out of this work came several articles on urban demography that analyzed the differential distribution and concentrations of older people in North American cities. The frequency with which I found high concentrations of older people in the core areas of central cities led others to label them "gray ghettoes."

Recently, I returned to this area of research only to find the tendency to concentrate (or to segregate them, if you will) had increased dramatically during the 1950s, and then slowed during the 1960s. If the 1980 census data ever arrives, I will be able to continue my comparison of age concentration between cities of high and low growth rates.

In 1959, I was baptized and became a "gerontologist." The ceremony took place in Berkeley, California, after I—along with forty other Fellows from all parts of the country—had spent one month in an intensive training session labeled the "Inter-University Institute of Social Gerontology." Guided by such pioneers and prophets as Wilma Donahue, Clark Tibbetts, Ernest Burgess, and Robert Havighurst, we learned our catechism and were duly ordained as gerontologists. Among the cadre of graduates of the Institute during its two summers of operation were such notables as Juanita Kreps, Arnold Rose, Irving Rosow, Leonard Breen, and Albert Wessen. Each of us wound up carving out a sphere of interests.

One of *my* continuing preoccupations as a gerontologist has been the demography of aging, particularly the measurement and analysis of changes in age composition of populations as they experience the drastic reductions of death rates and birth rates that are inherent aspects of modern times. For several decades I was content with rather straightforward description of information about the process.

Recently, annoyed by misinterpretations and erroneous conclusions from these data, I have become somewhat polemical. It is one thing to describe and acknowledge the facts of demographic aging, that is, that the percentage of the population 65 and over has increased from less than 3 percent in 1870 to more than 11 percent at the present time; it is quite another to treat this salubrious trend as a burdensome problem, portending economic disaster.

Recognizing the political motivations behind some of the misinterpretations, I recently resurrected a paper that I had given in 1978 in Tokyo under the neutral title, "Demographic Aging and Economic Dependency" and changed it to "Can We Afford Our Aging Populations?" Briefly the arguments are as follows: although our population is certainly aging and the ratio of elderly people to the labor force is rising, this emphatically does not mean that our total dependency load is increasing. On the contrary, because of falling birth rates and declining child populations that more than offset the increased numbers of the aged, the total dependency ratios are going down. We have fewer dependent persons per worker in the United States than we had a century ago, and modernized countries characteristically have decisively lower dependency loads than less developed countries. With our vastly greater resources, we certainly can afford our aging populations.

But this is just the most recent version in history of treating old age as a social problem. Most early gerontologists attached a negative value to old age. Stuart Queen, my former mentor, even treated it as a "social pathology" along with poverty, unemployment, mental illness, and even venereal disease. He is now 91 and appears to have found old age to be not all that bad!

This imagery continues. Recently, I received a request to give a guest lecture on the intriguing topic, "Aging as a Social Disease." I stalled momentarily, trying to determine whether the caller was serious. She was! And apparently she was not even aware of what an advanced case I was! I am almost sorry I didn't accept the invitation. Perhaps I could have learned something of the epidemiology of the ailment. On the other hand, there might have been some risk of personal embarrassment, since I understand that in registering a case of a social disease, one is required to identify his contact and I'm not sure where I caught it!

The stereotype of old age as a period of physiological and psychological deterioration received sociological justification from the so-called disengagement theory. Based upon the Kansas City Study of Adult Life, and first published in 1960, disengagement theory was the sociological counterpart of the biological view that aging brings necessary physiological deterioration and the psychological view that there are parallel declines in perception, memory, and cognition. This theory stated that, from a sociological perspective, aging was a normal and necessary process of disengagement whereby the individual withdrew from the major roles of life while society, concomitantly, ceased to depend upon the individual for the performance of those roles. Thus, aging was viewed as a kind of social metabolism in which individuals—having served their function—dropped out and were replaced. The process was presented as a normal, natural, functional process which was necessary, and desired by both the individual and society. From the standpoint of the individual, successful aging was seen as graceful withdrawal from life. From the standpoint of society, it was the necessary extrusion of worn out parts.

There was an immediate and vociferous reaction to this point of view. Not only was it evident that this provided a naturalistic, scientific rationale for the new twentieth-century practice of retirement from the labor force, but it also had much broader implications for personal life styles and therapeutic practices. It justified the rocking chair life style. It excused custodial treatment. It flew in the face of the activist North American frontier "die-with-your-boots-on" philosophy. It had the potential of becoming a self-fulfilling prophecy, leading to much "rusting out" through rationalized inactivity.

Much gerontological research during the past two decades, including a bit of my own, has sought to test this theory, and it has emerged somewhat battered and misshapen. In a very trenchant critique of its status in 1975, Arlie Hochschild pointed out the following shortcomings: (1) the theory as originally stated could not be disproven, since all deviations could be explained away as unsuccessful disengagers, off in timing, élite exceptions, or variations in form; (2) disengagement is an omnibus term covering many different kinds of roles and relationships: cessation of one role does not necessarily portend withdrawal from others; (3) roles and relationships have different meanings to different people: they vary between cultures, they vary by social class and sex within societies. Disengagement from a work role may, for some, mean more time to spend with family; to some this may be a dreaded retreat; to others, an exciting adventure.

In summary, while there is a tendency in modernized societies to encourage disengagement from significant societal roles, most especially from employment, this is certainly not a uniform process. Some people disengage; others do not. People disengage from some roles while intensifying their engagement in other realms of life. There is no predictable uniformity about the time when people will disengage or from what roles; whether this is a permanent or temporary disengagement; or what it means to the individual concerned. We cannot, that is, say that there is a general disengagement process. We *can* say that the older generation at any given time is more diverse and *heterogeneous* than all younger age categories. They have had a greater variety of experiences and a wider range of backgrounds.

Another issue of social gerontology that I have wrestled with is the theory that modernization as a historical process results in lowering the status of the elderly in society. This was the theme of my book *Aging and Modernization*, coauthored with Lowell Holmes in 1972. It was stated in a more elaborate and systematic form in an article in 1974. It has been debated and researched by historians, economists, anthropologists, and sociologists. As data has accumulated, pro and con, I have been motivated toward another critique and evaluation of the theory.

At the present juncture I should judge that the status of the theory, in a much simplified form, is about as follows: (1) The relative status of the aged in North America did decline between 1770 and 1950 (this transcends the disagreement between two eminent historians as to the precise time and the reasons for the change); (2) There has been a reversal of that trend within the United States, dating from about 1960. All social indicators show that the welfare and status of the elderly in the United States have moved upward since that time; (3) The lumping together of all premodern, that is, preindustrial societies, was unjustified. While Leo Simmons in his classical work on *The Role of the Aged in Primitive Societies* did extol the status of the aged in the 71 societies included in that study, it is clear now that that was an overgeneralization, hinted at even in his work by cases that were treated as exceptions. In the light of subsequent work, it appears probable that the status of the aged was highly variable in collective hunting and fishing economies. In such societies it appears that the elderly shared the abundance during times of plenty but were among the first denied in times of severe scarcity; (4) The decline in the status of the elderly in modern societies may more properly be seen as the rise in status of the young as a part of the democratization of society. In agrarian societies, in which elderly males controlled land and inheritance rights, elders may have had high status through power and not necessarily love. When the predominant economic activities shifted from the home (or farm) to the factory (or city) and when work and productivity became an individual matter rather than a community or family matter, the elderly tended to lose out in the competition; (5) Modernization is not a uniform or unidirectional process; the statement of a theory using it as the independent variable must account for different directions, speeds and patterns of social change, as well as somewhat different arrival points or destinations within a world system.

In summary, I have sought to discuss some of the trends, current issues, and problems of the new and burgeoning field of social geron- tology. I have touched on the demographic trends and their misinter- pretation. I have cited the checkered history of disengagement theory, and reviewed my engagement with modernization theory as it relates to aging. I would like to note that I have no intention of disengaging from the intellectual issues with which I have been concerned, a few of which I have discussed today. In fact, it is probable that I shall devote more of my time and energies to writing and research related to them. If I have been unduly autobio- graphical, I hope you will forgive me. This is the first time I have ever retired. With practice, I might do it with more grace and finesse.

An Informal Dialogue

QUESTION ONE: Regarding your theory of modernization and the declining status of the aged, do you mean to imply that the aged in our country are worse off now than they used to be?
ANSWER: Not at all. The modernization theory distinguishes be- tween the relative and absolute status of the aged. It is probable that the elderly and other age groups in our society have, in an absolute sense, greater economic security and a better standard of living than their counterparts in preindustrial societies. This is not to belittle the plight of poverty-stricken elderly in an affluent society. My point concerns the *relative* status of the aged. The prestige and honor of the elderly compared with younger age groups has declined. Their dis- advantage is more psychological than life-threatening. It is, nonethe- less, painful and humiliating. I should reiterate that the relative status of the aged has increased somewhat since 1960. But we must in the future readdress the real targets and concerns of society—pover- ty, disease, hunger, loneliness, and so on. Aging has some affinity with these conditions, but aging is not the disease, either social or physical. These real problems of society must be brought back into

focus, and the elderly encompassed within each of them must receive attention, but this is not because they are elderly, but because they are poor, ill, hungry, lonely, or whatever.

QUESTION TWO: In light of the criticisms which you and others made against it, why do you think disengagement theory received *any* support?

ANSWER: The image of the disengagement of older people tends to be confirmed and reinforced by the employment of methodologies that render distorted views of reality. Cross-sectional studies comparing different age groups at the same point in time are the usual basis for generalizations about the effects of aging. But such studies inevitably confound the effects of aging with the effects of different experiences of different age cohorts. For example, people who are over 65 years old today have personally experienced two World Wars and the Great Depression. The generations born after 1945 have not had those experiences. Any residual effects of those experiences will show up as differences between people 65 and over and those under 35. But the differences are not due to age. Many of the real or imagined *problems* of the aged, such as poverty, ill-health, lower mental acuity, inactivity, isolation, may derive in part from less educational opportunities, different work experience, rural background, poorer health care, and different diets of people who were children during the first quarter of the century. When the activities of older people are studied *longitudinally,* as with the later follow-up studies of the Kansas City Study of Adult Life, the activity patterns usually discovered involve a continuity with that person's previous style of life. Those who were not involved in many social activities at mid-life don't retire to become social climbers; those who have been active, barring health or resource limitations, tend to remain engaged in their later lives.

QUESTION THREE: Could you tell us some of *your* plans for remaining engaged?

ANSWER: I did mention my desire to continue my writing and research, particularly on cross-cultural differences in aging. I intend to read some things I have had waiting on my shelves. If I ever have time, there are numerous works I want to re-read, such as, for example, Thorstein Veblen's *Theory of the Leisure Class*. This time I shall be reading it with questions in mind: how could such a penetrating mind—even as a professor at the University of Missouri in the early 1900s—have failed to forecast the development of a new leisure class, far different from the idle rich of whom he was writing—the elderly retired who were just becoming a statistical entity in our society?

At the same time, I expect to bring some kind of culmination to a hobby I have pursued for 45 years. The year 1982 was the 300th anniversary of the migration of the Cowgill family along with other Quaker families, under the leadership of William Penn, to these United States. I feel the compulsion to provide some kind of public record of these 45 years of play (research) in honor of this anniversary.

Finally, there are other areas of life and experience—intellectual and geographic—which I want to experience, but I also want with T.V. Smith to "savor the unassessable joys of inactivity." If I am also able to disengage myself sufficiently from current problems and responsibilities, perhaps I can feel relief from the pressure to provide answers to questions for which there are no known answers, and to give advice on issues for which human experience provides no precedents.

Bibliography

Association of American Medical Colleges. *Proceedings of the Regional Institutes on Geriatrics and Medical Education,* 1983.

Beard, W. J., Kalau, E. I., & Nobach, R. K. "Geriatric Education in a Nursing Home." *The Gerontologist* 23 (2):1983, pp. 132–135.

Brown, G. W., & Harris, T. *Social Origins of Depression: A Study of Psychiatric Disorder in Women.* New York: Macmillan, 1978.

Carboni, D. *Geriatric Medicine in the United States and Great Britain.* Westport, CT: Greenwood Press, 1982.

Champion, E. W., & Goldman, M. "The Rehabilitation Needs of Elderly Medical Patients." *Clinical Research* 29 (1981): 499–503.

Dans, P. E., & Kerr, M. R. "Gerontology and Geriatrics in Medical Education." *New England Journal of Medicine* 300 (1979): 228–232.

Devitt, M., & Checkoway, B. "Participation in Nursing Home Residents Councils: Promise and Practice." *The Gerontologist* 22 (February, 1982), pp. 49–53.

Diamond, T. "Nursing Homes as Trouble." *Urban Life* (October, 1983), pp. 1–23.

Dobrof, R., Metsch, J., & Moody, H. R. "The Long-Term Care Challenge: Rationalizing a Continuum of Care for Chronically Impaired Elderly." *Mt. Sinai J. Med.* 47 (1980): 387–395.

Evashwick, C. "Long-term Care Becomes Major New Role for Hospitals." *Hospitals* 56 (1982): 50–55.

Freeland, M. S., & Schendler, C. E. "National Health Expenditure Growth in the 1980's: An Aging Population, New Technologies, and Increasing Competition." *Health Care Financing Review* 4 (March, 1983).

Fry, C. L., et al. *Dimensions: Aging, Culture, and Health.* New York: J. F. Bergin Publishers, 1981.

Fry, C. L., & Keith, J. *New Methods for Old Age Research.* Chicago: Center for Urban Policy, 1980.

Gustafson, D., Fiss, C., Fryback, J., Smelser, P., & Hiles, M. "Quality of Care in Nursing Homes: The New Wisconsin Evaluation System." *Long-Term Care Administration* 9:2 (Summer, 1981), pp. 40–55.

Haug, M. R. (ed.). *Elderly Patients and Their Doctors.* New York: Springer Publishing Company, 1981.

Ingman, S. R., Lawson, I. R., & Carboni, D. "Medical Direction in Long-Term Care." *J. of Amer. Ger. Society* 26 (1978): 157–166.

Ingman, S. R., McDonald, C. A., & Lusky, R. "An Alternative Model in Geriatric Care." *J. of Amer. Ger. Society* 26 (1979): 279–283.

Ingman, S. R., & Lawson, I. R. "Utilization of Specialized Ambulatory Care by the Elderly: A Study of a Clinic." *Med. Care* 20 (1982): 331–338.

Kane, R. A., & Kane, R. L. *Assessing the Elderly: A Practical Guide to Management.* Lexington, MA: Lexington Books, 1981.

Kane, R. L., & Kane, R. A. *Value Preferences and Long Term Care.* Lexington, MA: D.C. Heath, 1982.

Kausler, D. H. *Experimental Psychology and Human Aging.* New York: John Wiley & Sons, 1982.

Koff, T. H. *Long-Term Care: An Approach to Serving the Frail Elderly.* Boston: Little, Brown & Co., 1982.

Kutza, E. A. *The Benefits of Old Age: Social-Welfare Policy for the Elderly.* Chicago: University of Chicago Press, 1981.

Olsen, L. P. "A Nurse Administered Long-Term Care Unit." *J. of Gerontological Nursing* 6 (October, 1980), pp. 616–21.

Quadagno, J. S. (ed.). *Aging, the Individual, & Society: Readings in Social Gerontology.* New York: St. Martin's Press, 1980.

Rabin, D. L. "Physician Care in Nursing Homes." *Annals of Internal Medicine* 94 (1981): 126–128.

Rango, N. "Nursing-Home Care in the United States." *New England Journal of Medicine* 307, Vol. 14, Sept. 30, 1982, pp. 883–889.

Rubenstein, L. Z., Rhee, L., & Kane, R. L. "The Role of Geriatric Assessment Unit in Caring for the Elderly: An Analytic Review." *J. of Gerontology* 37 (September, 1982), pp. 513–521.

Russell, L. B. "An Aging Population and the Use of Medical Care." *Med. Care,* June 1981, pp. 633–43.

Simmons, V., Fittipaldi, L., Holovet, E., Mones, P., Gerardi, R., & Mech, A. "Assessing the Quality of Care in Skilled Nursing Homes." *Long-Term Care Administration,* 9:2 (1981), pp. 1–17.

Sohngen, M., & Smith, R. J. "Image of Old Age in Poetry." *The Gerontologist* (April, 1978), pp. 181–186.

Spicker, S. F., & Gadow, S. (eds.). *Nursing: Images and Ideals—Opening Dialogue with the Humanities.* New York: Springer Publishing Company, 1980.

Smith, D. B. *Long-Term Care in Transition: The Regulation of Nursing Homes.* Washington, D.C.: AUPHA Press, 1981.

Solomon, R. "Aging Individuals in Long-Term Care Need Choice and Autonomy." *Generations* 5:3 (Spring, 1981), pp. 32–38.

Soski, C. W. "Teaching Nursing Home Staff about Patients' Rights." *The Gerontologist* 21 (August, 1981), pp. 424–430.

Index